AF333857

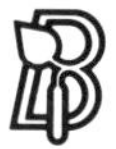

AAS
Agents and Actions Supplements
Vol. 30

Series Editor
K. Brune, Erlangen

Birkhäuser Verlag
Basel · Boston · Berlin

Inflammatory Indices in Chronic Bronchitis

Edited by

Carl G. A. Persson
Ralph Brattsand
Lauri A. Laitinen
Per Venge

1990

Birkhäuser Verlag
Basel · Boston · Berlin

Volume Editor's Addresses:

Carl G. A. Persson
Department of Clinical Pharmacology
University Hospital of Lund
S–221 85 Lund/Sweden

Ralph Brattsand
Laboratory of Pharmacology
Research & Development Department
AB Draco
Box 34
S–221 00 Lund/Sweden

Lauri A. Laitinen
Department of Explorative Clinical Research
AB Draco
Box 34
S–221 00 Lund/Sweden

Per Venge
Laboratory for Inflammation Research
Department of Clinical Chemistry
University Hospital
S–751 85 Uppsala/Sweden

Deutsche Bibliothek Cataloging-in-Publication Data

Inflammatory indices in chronic bronchitis / ed. by Carl G. A.
Persson ... – Basel ; Boston ; Berlin : Birkhäuser, 1990
   (Agents and actions : Supplements ; Vol. 30)
   ISBN 3-7643-2370-1 (Basel ...)
   ISBN 0-8176-2370-1 (Boston)
NE: Persson, Carl G. A. [Hrsg.]; Agents and actions / Supplements

TABLE OF CONTENTS

FOREWORD

Epidemiological studies of Chronic Bronchitis/ Chronic Obstructive Airway Disease (CB/COAD) have demonstrated that hypersecretory glandular activity, as well as infections, are not the most important risk factors determining the serious decline in lung function in this disease. Instead, inflammatory indices are emerging as characteristic features of the pathology and pathophysiology of CB/COAD. It is possible that continuous inflammatory processes cause structural changes and thus provide the anatomical basis for airway obstruction which, once established, is only partly reversible.

We felt it was timely to gather leading international researchers who could provide critical updates on CB/COAD, its pathology and clinical/ experimental assessments. The latter aspect included not only the fundamentals of airway function but also, and in greater detail, cellular and solute indices which can now be used to determine inflammation in CB/COAD. The meeting was made possible by a grant from Draco/Astra (Sweden and Finland). We particularly acknowledge the expert assistance of Mrs. Eva Engberg in all facets of the present work.

CB/COAD remains a major public health problem. It is a common cause for early retirement and is one of the fastest rising causes of death in many countries. We hope that the material collected in this book will provide a momentum to research interests into basic aspects of CB/COAD and, perhaps more importantly, into therapeutic interventions. Indeed, these two interests need not be divided. Significant lessons would be learned about the disease from studies of the effect of anti-inflammatory drug treatment on the annual decline in lung function in CB/COAD, especially if select inflammatory indices are monitored as well.

Carl Persson, Ralph Brattsand, Lauri Laitinen, Per Venge

1) AIRWAY PATHOLOGY OF FUNCTIONAL SIGNIFICANCE IN CHRONIC BRONCHITIS AND CHRONIC OBSTRUCTIVE AIRWAY DISEASE

J.C. Hogg

University of British Columbia, St. Paul's Hospital
1081 Burrard Street, Vancouver, B.C., Canada V6Z 1Y6

SUMMARY: The three major hypothesis for reduction in the calibre of the peripheral airways in chronic obstructive lung disease are 1) a loss of elastic recoil in the alveolar supporting structure, 2) destruction of the alveolar attachments to the outer wall of the small airways, and 3) a chronic inflammatory process in the wall and lumen of the peripheral airways. This presentation is based on the analysis of an ongoing study where lung function has been measured a few days prior to lung resection. The data collected to date support the third hypothesis and are of interest in developing strategies to treat patients with COAD because they suggest that therapy should be directed at preventing the inflammatory process in the peripheral airways rather than the prevention of lung destruction by emphysema.

INTRODUCTION

The development of a reliable method of measuring distal bronchial pressure (Macklem & Mead, 1967) allowed the direct measurement of peripheral airways resistance in human lungs obtained at autopsy (Hogg et al., 1968). These studies (Hogg et al., 1968) showed that in normal lungs, the resistance of peripheral bronchi and bronchioles smaller than 2 mm in diameter was much less than that in the larger airways. It also showed that the peripheral airways smaller than 2 mm in diameter were the major site of increased resistance in obstructive lung disease. Since then, there has been disagreement over the exact distribution of airways resistance in normal lungs (Niewoehner & Kleinerman, 1974; Hoppin et al., 1978; Van Brabandt et al., 1983) and the old problem about how much of this increase in pressure is related to tissue viscance has been reintroduced. However, all of the studies known to us have concluded that the peripheral airways are the site of increased resistance in obstructive lung disease and the work done that is to be presented here is based on that hypothesis.

There are three possible mechanisms for this increase in peripheral airways resistance in disease. One is that the loss of lung elastic recoil caused by emphysema allows the airways to narrow (Butler et al., 1960; Petty et al., 1984). The second is that they narrow because the alveolar attachments which provide their support are destroyed by the emphysematous process (Dayman, 1951; Petty et al., 1986; Saetta et al., 1985), and the third is that an inflammatory process in the airway wall and lumen disorganizes peripheral airway structure and function to increase resistance (Hogg et al., 1968; McLean, 1957; McLean, 1958).

The hypothesis that airways narrow because of either decreased elastic recoil or destroyed alveolar attachments was not supported by the retrograde catheter studies (Hogg et al., 1968). If decreased elastic recoil had been the sole explanation for the increased resistance, it should have been possible to lower airways resistance towards normal values by inflating the lung and it was not. Similarly, if the increased resistance was due to destruction of the alveolar support by emphysema, the resistance should have been less with lung inflation than deflation (Dayman, 1951) and this did not happen either. Indeed, to make measurements of resistance, it is necessary to plot flow against the pressure drop from the catheter tip to the pleural surface and electrically subtract elastic recoil pressure to obtain flow resistive pressure. The resistance is the slope of the straight line formed by this relationship and these were the same on inflation and deflation in all cases as the lung was cycled over a small volume change at frequencies of up to 4 per second. Therefore, in our studies using direct measurements of peripheral airways pressures and flows (Hogg et al., 1968), we concluded that the problem in the peripheral airways was organic in nature and that it was most likely associated with a chronic inflammatory process in the airway wall and lumen. Although more recent (Petty et al., 1986; Saetta et al., 1985) studies have continued to emphasize the importance of elastic recoil changes and changes in the radial traction of small airways as contributing factors in the pathogenesis of the airways obstruction, our work has supported McLean's (McLean, 1956; 1957; 1958) earlier hypothesis that organic disease in the small airways is responsible for the airways obstruction.

The classic postmortem study of Niewoehner et al. (1974) was the first to show that cigarette smoking produced structural changes due to an inflammatory response in the peripheral airways. However, several studies indicate that the decline in function seen in COPD cannot be simply explained by smoking. Fletcher and his associates (Fletcher et al., 1976; Fletcher & Peto, 1977; Peto et al., 1984) showed that this excessive decline only occurs in about 20 % of heavy smokers which suggests the hypothesis that this abnormality in airways function must be linked to an excessive inflammatory reaction in the peripheral airways. Whether this excessive response is due to a more peripheral delivery of a similar dose of smoke, a genetic difference in the control of the inflammatory response, the presence of an extra stimulus such as latent viral infection in the peripheral airways or some other mechanism remains to be determined.

QUANTITATION OF THE INFLAMMATORY RESPONSE
IN PERIPHERAL AIRWAYS

When tissue covered by an epithelial surface is damaged, there is

an organized inflammatory response. Early in this response there
is an exudation of plasma and cells from the vascular space into
the tissue where the damage has occurred (Taussig, 1984; Florey,
1970). This activates proteins that normally remain in the
vascular space and potent mediators are generated from the
complement, kinin, coagulation and fibrinolytic systems. These
plasma-derived mediators, along with others, generated in the
tissue from mast cells, nerve endings and damaged cell membranes,
control the vascular exudative phenomena associated with the
inflammatory response. The structural changes that occur include
tissue swelling due to vascular congestion and fluid exudation
from the vessels into the interstitial space. The migration of
polymorphonuclear and mononuclear cells into the damaged area and
the organization of this exudate by vascular and connective
tissue elements is followed by a gradual return toward a normal
structure. In tissues covered by a mucous secreting epithelium
such as the airways, these changes are accompanied by a shedding
of epithelial cells and excess secretion of mucus (Florey, 1970).
This is associated with a replacement of the shed epithelium by
either squamous cells (squamous cell metaplasia) or goblet cells
(goblet cell metaplasia). In a chronic inflammatory process the
epithelium may either become hyperplastic or ulcers may form in
it if the defects are not properly repaired. There may also be an
increase in both the smooth muscle and collagen in the subepithelial tissue and scars may form in the damaged areas. This
leads to contraction in the damaged area and fixed narrowing of
the airway lumen.

The approach we have used to overcome the difficult problem of
quantitating the degree of change that occurs in damaged airways
(Cosio et al., 1978; Wright et al., 1984; Wright et al., 1985)
has been to use photographs of varying degrees of a particular
structural change to grade the response. This allowed each airway
in the histological sample obtained from the resected lung to be
examined and assigned a grade ranging between 0 (no change) and
3 (maximum change from normal). These grades are then expressed
as a percent of the maximum possible change which is the number

of airways examined times three. In an early study (Cosio et al., 1978), we assigned grades to the membranous airways less than 2 mm in diameter in each lung for the number of inflammatory cells present, the deposition of collagen, the amount of muscle in the airway wall, the degree of squamous cell and, goblet cell metaplasia, the presence of ulcers in the mucosa, the amount of pigment in the airway wall, the amount of exudate in the airway lumen. This total score for the inflammatory process which was then the sum of all of these individual scores was used to rank the cases.

These data (Cosio et al., 1978) showed that the changes that contributed to an increase in the total were consistent with what might be expected with a more extensive and severe inflammatory response in the peripheral airways. They included the presence of an increasing number of inflammatory cells, increased connective tissue deposition in the airway wall, epithelial metaplasia and ulceration in the mucosa. The data also showed that the increase in the score for the inflammatory process was associated with increased malfunction of the peripheral airways and a decline in the FEV_1/FVC ratio.

These observations were extended in a subsequent study of 96 additional cases (Wright et al., 1984) where the respiratory bronchioles were also examined using a similar but slightly different grading system to estimate the inflammatory process in these airways. In this study, the cases were divided on the basis of the observed FEV_1 which ranged from 100 % predicted to <60 % predicted and showed that there was a good correlation between several of the markers of the inflammatory response and the decrease in FEV_1. These findings have been supported by studies from other laboratories using the same set of pictures to grade the airways (Saetta et al., 1985; Berend et al., 1981).

It is very important to understand that the changes that were graded represent histological markers of the inflammatory response that may not in themselves be responsible for any abnormality in airways function. For example, we have no measure of the mediators released in the tissue, the volume of fluid exudation or the amount of protein in it. We also do not know the changes in tension that may have occurred in the airways surface that could easily account for airways narrowing in the early stages of the process. Therefore, to determine if the inflammatory process could really account for the changes in airways function that occurred, we carried out a series of animal experiments. In this study (Baile et al., 1982) a mild inflammatory response was produced in the airways by exposing them to an aerosol of weak acid with lung function being measured before and after the exposure. A control group exposed to saline was included and the animals were sacrificed and the airways examined after the functional studies were complete. The results showed that the inflammatory response in the airways was responsible for a decrease in peripheral airways function. Taking the human and animal results together, it seemed reasonable to conclude that there is a chronic inflammatory response in the peripheral airways of patients with airway obstruction and that the progression of this response provided a reasonable structural basis for the deterioration in airways function.

EMPHYSEMA

The fact that emphysema is present in the lungs of people who smoke is very well established (Snider et al., 1985), and these lesions are thought to be due to dilatation and destruction of respiratory bronchioles by a functional protease imbalance (Snider et al., 1985). The extent and severity of this lesion in resected lungs can be estimated using a modification of a picture grading system developed by Thurlbeck et al. (1970). That has been validated for the study of surgically resected lungs (Wright et al., 1986). Using this procedure we have been able to show (Hogg et al., 1989) the relationship between the emphysematous process and the fall in FEV_1 was due to the lesions becoming more prevalent rather than more severe. This evidence that the severity of the macroscopic emphysema is not associated with lowering of the FEV_1 does not support the concept that emphysema is an important cause of airways obstruction.

Very recently Wright et al. (1988) extended these studies by quantitating the degree of peribronchiolar support in smokers and non-smokers. Their results confirmed those of Saetta et al. (1985) in showing that smoking is associated with an increased inflammatory response in the peripheral airways as well as destruction of the alveoli supporting the small airways. Surprisingly, when the smokers who had macroscopic emphysema were compared to those who did not, there was no difference in the severity of the destruction of the alveolar attachments between the two groups. These data suggest that macroscopic emphysema and destruction of alveoli supporting bronchioles occur as independent processes. Taken together, these results (Hogg et al., 1989; Wright et al., 1988) suggest that neither the severity of the emphysematous process estimated at the macroscopic level nor the destruction of the peribronchiolar support measured at the microscopic level is directly responsible for the airways narrowing.

CONCLUSION: Our work suggests that the airways obstruction that develops in about 20 % of heavy smokers is not caused by a loss of elastic recoil in the alveolar supporting network (Hogg et al., 1968), the destruction of the peribronchiolar alveolar support (Wright et al., 1988) or the presence of macroscopic emphysematous lung destruction (Hogg et al., 1989). Our working hypothesis is that the obstruction is related to encroachment on the lumen of the small airways produced a chronic inflammatory process in the wall of the distal airways. The importance of establishing whether or not the hypothesis is correct is that treatments designed to reverse an inflammatory response in the peripheral airways are likely to be very different than those designed to prevent the destruction of the alveolar surface by emphysema.

Acknowledgement: Supported by the Medical Research Council of Canada, the British Columbia Lung Association, and the Tobacco Manufacturers' Council of Canada

DISCUSSION

Arborelius. The most important variable, transpulmonary pressure, was missing in your presentation. Was there a relation between elastic recoil pressure and emphysema score?

Hogg. I did not show the data but there is no difference in elastic recoil between the patients with obstruction and those without obstruction.

Pride. Is the wall thickening less significant in large than in small airways? The mean thickening seemed if anything to be greater in large airways but presumably this was based on fewer samples according for the wider confidence limits in large airways.

Hogg. Data is more convincing for bronchioles than for bronchi because there are fewer bronchi in the sample.

Brattsand. What is known about small airway inflammation in α_1-antitrypsin deficiency induced emphysema? Can this experiment of nature help in elucidating the relation between alveolar and small airway inflammation?

Hogg. This needs to be studied. I would guess that many of the α_1-antitrypsin deficient people have emphysema but only those who also have an inflammatory process in the peripheral airways have airways obstruction.

Persson. In your study you indicated that loss of elastic recoil was not an explanation for the baseline obstruction. My comment is that when you challenge airways with bronchoconstricting agents loss of elastic recoil would result in abnormally large contraction.

Annika Laitinen. Did you do more detailed analysis of the inflammatory infiltrate cells in the airways? Did you also see inflammatory cells in the microvessels in the bronchial mucosa?

Hogg. We are in the process of analyzing the cell population with monoclonal antibodies.

Arborelius. In the normal lung airways dilate in relation to increase in lung volume. Is your message that inflamed, thick airways walls do not dilate in relation to increase in trans-pulmonary pressure - or that the compliance is decreased - which seems probable from your picture?

Hogg. The compliance of airways is difficult to measure. However there are disproportional measures for the trans-pulmonary pressure.

REFERENCES

Baile, E.M., Wright, J.L., Pare, P.D., and Hogg, J.C. (1982) 126, 298-301.
Berend, W., Wright, J.L., Thurlbeck, W.M., Markine, G.E., and Woolcock, A. (1981) Chest 79, 263-268.
Butler, J., Caro, C.G., Alcala, R., and Dubois, A.B. (1960) J. Clin. Invest. 39, 584-591.
Cosio, M.G., Ghezzo, H., Hogg, J.C., Corbin, R., Loveland, M., Dosman, J., and Macklem, P.T. (1978) New Engl. J. Med. 298, 1277-1281.
Dayman, H. (1951) J. Clin. Invest. 30, 1175-1190.
Fletcher, C., Peto, R., Tinker, C., and Speizer, F.E. (1976) Oxford University Press, Oxford.
Fletcher, C., and Peto, R. (1977) Brit. Med. J. 1, 1645-1648.
Florey, H.W. (1970) General Pathology. Lloyd-Luke, London. 4th Edition.
Hogg, J.C., Macklem, P.T., and Thurlbeck, W.M. (1968) New Engl. J. Med. 278, 1355-1360.
Hogg, J.C, Pare, P.D., and Wright, J.L. (1989) In: Bronchitis IV. (H.J. Sluiter and R. van der Lande, Eds) Van Gorcum,

ASSEN/Maastrecht. pp. 123-132.
Hoppin, F.G., Green, M., and Morgan, M. (1978) J. Appl. Physiol. 44, 728-37.
Macklem, P.T., and Mead, J. (1967) J. Appl. Physiol. 22, 395-401.
McLean, K.H. (1956) Australasian Ann. Med. 5, 254.
McLean, K.H. (1957) Australasian Ann. Med. 6, 29.
McLean, K.H. (1958) Am. J. Med. 25, 62-74.
Niewoehner, D.E., and Kleinerman, J. (1974) J. Appl. Physiol. 36, 412-418.
Niewoehner, D.E., Kleinerman, J., and Rice, D.B. (1974) New Engl. J. Med. 291, 755-758.
Peto, R., Speizer, F.E., Cochrane, A.L., Moore, F., Fletcher, C.M., Tinker, C.M., Higgins, I.T.T., Gray, R.G., Richards, S.M., Gilleland, J., and Roman-Smith, B. (1984) Am. Rev. Respir. Dis. 128, 491-500.
Petty, T.L., Silvers, G.W., and Stanford, R.E. (1984) Am. Rev. Respir. Dis. 130, 42-45.
Petty, T.L., Silvers, G.W., and Stanford, R.E. (1986) Am. Rev. Respir. Dis. 133, 132-135.
Saetta, M., Ghezzo, H., Kim, W.D., King, M., Angus, G.E., Wang, N-S., and Cosio, M. (1985) Am. Rev. Respir. Dis. 132, 894-900.
Snider, D.L., Kleinerman, J., Thurlbeck, W.M., and Bengali, Z. (1985) Am. Rev. Respir. Dis. 132, 182-185.
Taussig, M.J. (1984) Processes in pathology and microbiology. Blackwell Scientific Publications, Oxford. Second Edition.
Thurlbeck, W.M., Dunnill, M.S., Hartung, W., Heard, B.E., Hepplesten, A.G., and Lydin, R.C. (1970) Hum. Path. 1, 215-226.
Van Brabandt, H., Cauberghs, M., Verbeken, E., Moerman, P., Lauweryns, J.M., and van de Woestijne, K.P. (1983) J. Appl. Physiol. 55, 1733-1742.
Wright, J.L., Cosio, M.G., Wiggs, B., and Hogg, J.C. (1985) Arch. Path. Lab. Med. 109, 163-165.
Wright, J.L., Hobson, J.E., Wiggs, B., Pare, P.D., and Hogg, J.C. (1988) Lung 166, 277-286.
Wright, J.L., Lawson, L.M., Pare, P.D., Kennedy, S.M., Wiggs, B., and Hogg, J.C. (1984) Am. Rev. Respir. Dis. 129, 989-994.
Wright, J.L., Wiggs, B., Pare, P.D., and Hogg, J.C. (1986) Am. Rev. Respir. Dis. 133, 930-931.

2) ASSESSMENT OF LONG-TERM CHANGES IN AIRWAY FUNCTION

N.B. Pride

Department of Medicine, Royal Postgraduate Medical School
LONDON, W12 ONN, United Kingdom

SUMMARY: There is some evidence supporting long-term 'tracking' of decline in FEV_1 at least in middle-aged male smokers, so that a moderately reduced FEV_1 predicts subsequent disability and death. Distribution of individual rates of decline in FEV_1 stabilizes after follow-up for 4 to 5 years, but large and unexplained differences in decline in FEV_1 are found between individuals with similar smoking history. There are theoretical advantages to following post-bronchodilator FEV_1 but few studies of its usefulness are available. Changes in other tests derived from the single breath N_2 test or the maximum expiratory flow-volume curve have been less informative than originally postulated and their long-term prognostic value remains unknown.

INTRODUCTION

The dominant current theory of the evolution of chronic obstructive airway disease (COAD) in smokers is that proposed in the middle nineteen-seventies by Fletcher et al., (1976, 1977 [Fig. 1] Pathway A). In this paper I shall review current evidence for certain features of the natural history proposed by Fletcher and colleagues - particularly the insidious nature of the decline in lung function and the striking between-individual variability in susceptibility to the effects of cigarettes, so that less than 20 % of middle-aged male smokers develop severe, progressive airways obstruction. Factors which may contribute to the great variation in susceptibility between individuals are discussed in other chapters.

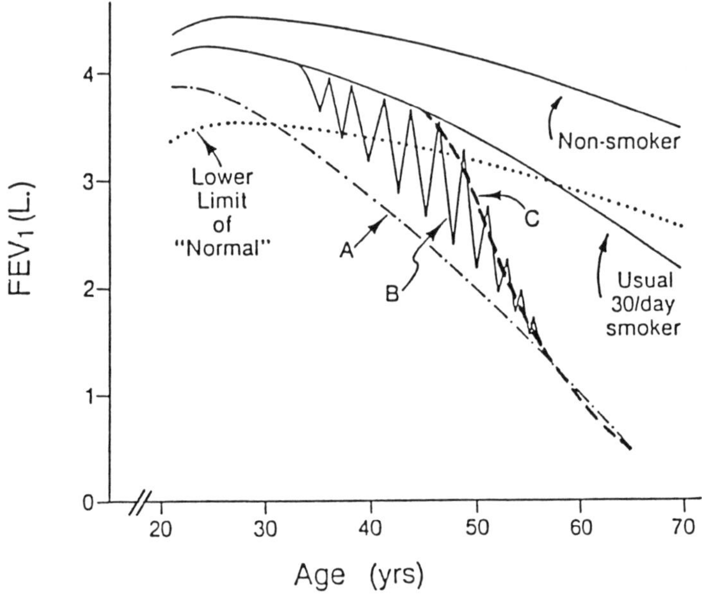

Figure 1. Three possible pathways (A,B,C) for development of disabling COAD. Changes in FEV$_1$ for an average healthy non-smoker, lower limit of normal FEV$_1$ and changes in the 'usual' smoker of 30 cigarettes/day are also shown.

Pathway A indicates the preclinical course suggested by Fletcher and colleagues (1976, 1977) with a moderately accelerated rate of decline in FEV$_1$ developing early in the course of smoking and sustained over many years.

Pathway B indicates a period of fluctuating FEV$_1$ ("chronic asthmatic bronchitis") preceding the development of severe irreversible reduction in FEV$_1$.

Pathway C remains indistinguishable from the 'usual' smoker until late middle age when there is a relatively brief period of rapid decline in FEV$_1$.

(Slightly modified from Fig. 3 in B. Burrows. An overview of obstructive lung disease. Med. Clin. N. America 1981; 65: 455-471).

ASSESSING RATES OF DECLINE IN FEV$_1$

The insidious development of COAD was first suggested by the modest increase in rates of decline in FEV$_1$ observed in symptomatic patients with COAD, but such selected groups cannot give a true picture of the natural history of smoking-related disease in the wider population. Subsequently Fletcher et al., (1976, 1977) obtained direct evidence of the early change in FEV$_1$ in working men in London; because they found a relationship between the annual rate of decline in FEV$_1$ over 8 years ("slope") and the level of FEV$_1$ they suggested smokers could be identified by reduction in FEV$_1$ by early middle age. This implies that individuals in the top or bottom percentiles with regard to FEV$_1$ have to stay in the same percentile over many subsequent years and show 'tracking' as has been described in longitudinal studies of blood pressure. In North America an alternative hypothesis has been popular. Because the initial stages of smoking-related lung damage are characterized by inflammatory and obstructive changes in the peripheral airways, which have an enormous functional reserve, these pathological changes may cause few symptoms and negligible decline in tests of overall lung function such as the FEV$_1$ until they become very severe and widespread. Thus susceptible smokers might only declare themselves by accelerated decline of FEV$_1$ over a relatively short number of years in late middle age, while earlier in their smoking years their FEV$_1$, though slightly lower than in most non-smokers, might be indistinguishable from the general population of smokers most of whom would be destined to follow a benign course (Fig. 1; pathway C). If this was the usual natural history it would be difficult to study risk factors and interventions by following annual decline in lung function, because studies early in the smoking lifetime would not be predictive of later disability, while studies in symptomatic subjects are complicated by exclusions due to severe disease and 'survivor' effects.

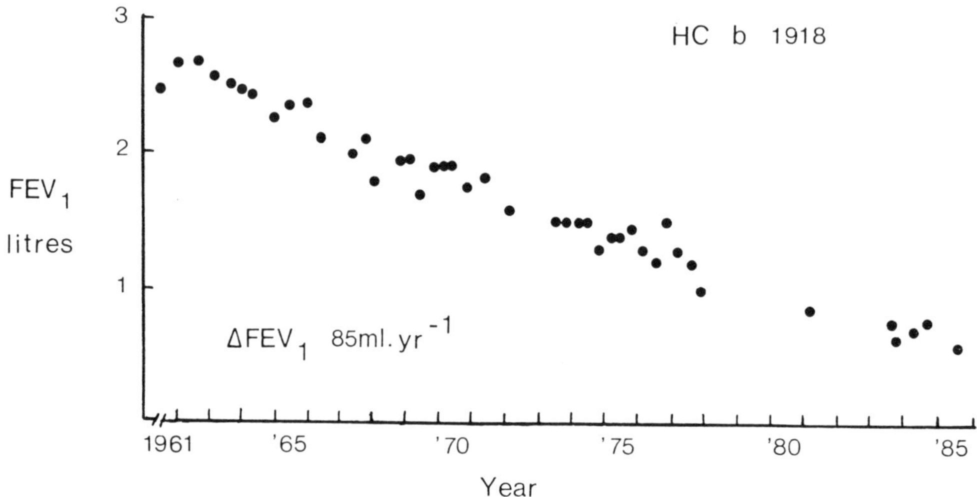

Figure 2. Change in pre-bronchodilator FEV$_1$ over 25 years in a male cigarette smoker.

Since Fletcher's original monograph some further studies have been made of the strength of 'tracking' of decline in lung function. Undoubtedly individual examples of relatively smooth decline over many years are found (Fig. 2); but the number of subjects whose detailed progress has been studied over sufficient years is relatively small. A 20 year follow-up study of 2718 men whose pulmonary function was assessed between 1954 and 1961 has supported 'tracking' indirectly, because the risk of death from chronic airflow obstruction was at least 50 times greater in men whose initial FEV$_1$ was more than 2 SD below average values than in men whose initial FEV$_1$ was above average (Peto et al., 1983). Most of these men were studied initially in middle age during their working life at a time when they had only minor abnormalities in FEV$_1$. Population studies in Tucson (Burrows et al., 1987), while confirming the presence of 'tracking' in middle aged males have not found it at other ages in men or at any age in women smokers, so that the overall strength of the tendency to tracking of lung function in the population remains uncertain.

There is a considerable error in estimating rates of decline in FEV_1 in an individual, due to the 'noise' produced by a mixture of true biological variation and measurement error. The longer the follow-up the greater the reliability of the estimate of true rate of decline in an individual subject. Alternatively a shorter follow-up with larger numbers allows group trends to be obtained. Burrows et al. (1986) have shown that the distribution of rates of decline stabilizes after about 4 or 5 years of follow-up. But even after this period of follow-up every study confirms the great between-individual variability of rate of decline in FEV_1. The reasons for this variability remain elusive. For intervention studies we wish to identify subjects likely to show rapid decline if untreated so that any effect of treatment is not too diluted by smokers with normal rates of decline whose subsequent course is not altered. Thus in our own studies, while on average current male cigarette smokers showed rather less than double the annual decline of FEV_1 found in healthy non-smokers - 47 ml/year compared to 26 ml/year - this average value concealed a considerable range of decline in FEV_1 in individuals, in particular a tail of smokers showing unusually rapid decline (Pride, 1985). In addition annual decline in FEV_1 in smokers possibly begins at a younger age than in healthy never-smokers, who show a plateau of FEV_1 until 30 to 35 years of age.

An obvious possible cause for the differing susceptibility of smokers is variation in exposure to tobacco smoke. When smokers are subdivided according to reported daily number of cigarettes smoked, a relation between cigarette numbers and annual decline in FEV_1 is found, but this relationship is relatively weak and a wide variation in annual rate of decline in FEV_1 persists among smokers of similar numbers of cigarettes. Characterization of smoking habit solely by current daily cigarette consumption - or even cumulative pack-years - does not allow for many other factors which influence the individual's exposure to cigarette smoke - such as the extent to which smoke is taken from the burning cigarette and inhaled deep into the lungs and the yield of tar, nicotine and other constituents of the cigarette. We have examined the relation between other aspects of smoking habit and decline in lung function in our own laboratory studies. Merely substituting occasional chemical markers of smoking such as breath carbon monoxide or blood cotinine levels for reported number of cigarettes smoked did not obviously strengthen the relation between smoking intensity and rate of decline in FEV_1. Comparison of the details of smoking pattern in small, but matched, groups of men showing either rapid or normal rates of decline in FEV_1 failed to show any significant differences. Reduction in the tar content of the cigarettes smoked had at most only a small effect in slowing the progression of airflow obstruction; any potential benefit may be counteracted by more intense smoking of low-tar cigarettes (Pride, 1985). Because there are so many potentially toxic constituents of tobacco smoke, it is impossible to exclude the possibility that some particular component of smoke, which might not be inhaled in parallel with any of the established markers, might be of overwhelming importance. But despite inevitable deficiencies in quantifying smoke exposure, I suspect there is probably a true wide difference in susceptibility between smokers which is not explained by variation in dose of tobacco smoke.

Population characteristics which are associated with accelerated decline are increasing age and, at least in the United Kingdom, lower socio-economic status. There are suggestions that men are more susceptible to airways obstruction than women but this is not found in all studies.

Although there are small improvements in lung function on stopping smoking in younger subjects with relatively minor loss of lung function, in longer-term studies in middle-aged or older subjects most evidence suggests that on stopping smoking there is little or no recovery of lung function but that subsequent rates of decline approach those found in never-smokers. Thus when assessed in terms of total "pack-years" (average daily consumption in packs of 20 cigarettes x years of smoking) it is not possible to distinguish between current smokers and ex-smokers. These observations support the hypothesis that lung function at a given time in an individual represents the cumulative effect of the total smoking history. Consequently the effect of any modification of smoking habit on baseline lung function is outweighed for many years by the cumulative earlier history and will take a lengthy period to be demonstrated by changes in mortality from chronic obstructive pulmonary disease. However, measuring prospective rates of decline of lung function will show immediate changes and a reasonable working hypothesis is that any anti-inflammatory intervention is unlikely to have larger effects on subsequent decline in lung function than giving up smoking.

Table I. Mean values for annual decline in men according to smoking status from longitudinal studies

	Age* (yrs)	ΔFEV_1 (ml/yr) Never-smokers	Current smokers Light	Heavy	Ex-smokers
Bande et al.	(1980)	18–56 27	30	39	
Huhti & Ikkala	(1980)	40–64 27	35		27
Beaty et al.	(1984)	20–60[+] 30		41	
Camilli et al.	(1987)	50–70 19		40	22
Dockery et al.	(1988)	50 35		42	35
Peat et al.	(1989)	40 32	41	43	
Peat et al.	(1989)	50 37	48	48	
Peat et al.	(1989)	60 41	50	53	

* Age indicates either range over which values were derived or figures for a standard age

Earlier reports of annual decline in FEV_1 in male smokers and non-smokers from longitudinal studies were summarized in the papers of Kauffman et al. (1979) and Bande et al. (1980). Some results in men reported in the 1980s from Finland (Huhti & Ikkala, 1980), USA (Camilli et al., 1987; Dockery et al., 1988) and Australia (Peat et al., 1989) are briefly summarized in Table I. All these studies also report results in women, which are not shown. The studies generally agree in showing that annual decline in FEV_1 accelerates with increasing age in both smokers and never-smokers and that rates of decline in FEV_1 in ex- smokers are close to those in never-smokers, but there is not clear agreement on whether male smokers are on average more susceptible to accelerated decline in lung function than women and even whether differences between smokers and healthy never-smokers increase with increasing age.

USE OF OTHER SPIROMETRIC INDICES OR OTHER TESTS OF LUNG FUNCTION TO ASSESS NATURAL HISTORY OF SMOKING-RELATED AIRWAYS OBSTRUCTION

In routine spirometry slow vital capacity is often measured as well as FEV_1; sometimes these measurements are repeated after bronchodilator treatment. In groups of men from whom those with asthma or on regular bronchodilator treatment have been excluded, we have found little difference in annual rates of decline in pre- or post-bronchodilator FEV_1. However there are potential advantages in using decline in post-bronchodilator FEV_1 as the primary measurement when subjects with some asthmatic features or on bronchodilator treatment are included as there is then less dependence on unsupervised withdrawal of treatment in the hours before measurement. Initial measurements of vital capacity (VC) are useful to establish that a reduced FEV_1 is associated with a reduced FEV_1/VC ratio, but as airway disease becomes established we have found that in many subjects there is much greater and erratic variation in VC than in FEV_1; hence we have persisted with pre- and post-bronchodilator FEV_1 as our main indicators of

decline in lung function, usually correcting for subject size by
dividing the values by height cubed, although others have used
height squared.

Table II. Value of single breath N_2 test for identifying the
high-risk smoker

	No. of subjects	Length of follow-up (years)
<u>Beaty et al.</u>, Am. Rev. Respir. Dis., 1984; 129: 660-667		
"only closing capacity at initial visit was consistently associated with subsequent loss of FEV_1 .... but only accounted for a modest proportion of the total variation seen in this sample"	805 men 669 women	4.7
<u>Olofsson et al.</u>, Eur. J. Respir. Dis., 1986; 69: 46-56.		
"An increase in the slope of phase III from 1.0 to 4.0 % N_2/l in moderate smokers was found to predict an increase in the rate of decline in FEV_1 by 50 %"	460 men	7
<u>Stanescu et al.</u>, Am. Rev. Respir. Dis., 1987; 135: 585-590.		
"sensitive tests do not permit identification of smokers at high risk"	850 men	6
<u>Buist et al.</u>, Am. Rev. Respir. Dis., 1988; 137: 293-301		
"single breath N_2 test can be useful in identifying the smoker who is at risk of developing chronic airflow limitation. However, its usefulness is diminished by the high proportion of smokers who have mild functional abnormalities but do not progress to develop chronic airflow limitation"	734 men & women	9-11

When the enormous functional reserve of the peripheral airways was appreciated in the nineteen-sixties, some scepticism developed as to the value of following FEV_1 for studying the pre-clinical stages of disease and for detecting smokers at risk of developing progressive airway obstruction. Furthermore 'low normal' values of FEV_1 are derived from a mixture of subjects whose lungs are structurally normal but smaller than average and others in whom disease has caused a decline in lung function from initial average or even above average values. Tests of lung function which are more sensitive to minor changes in the peripheral airways, such as the single breath N_2 test or the later part of the maximum expiratory flow-volume curve, should in theory therefore be useful both in their own right and as an aid to the interpretation of slightly reduced values in FEV_1. Unfortunately while several published studies support this hypothesis, there is a general consensus that the predictive value of the single breath N_2 test is not as strong as originally hoped (Table II).

In our own laboratory we have found similarly a disappointing predictive value of the single breath N_2 test; in particular we have not found an increasing divergence between smokers and never-smokers over the years of follow-up. We have also examined changes in the pre and postbronchodilator maximum expiratory flow-volume curve over a five-year follow-up period in some detail (Osmanliev et al., 1988). Most of the possible measurements (one and three second FEV, maximum flow rates at different %VC and transit time analysis) were analyzed. In male smokers aged more than 40 years at start of follow-up, decline in FEV_1 gave as strong a signal as any other measurement. As with the single breath N_2 test, there was no tendency for longitudinal changes in maximum expiratory flow rates to be larger in smokers than in never-smokers, although smokers had lower flow rates at recruitment. In male smokers less than 40 years old we still found some acceleration of annual decline in FEV_1 but the difference between smokers and non-smokers was smaller so there may be a place for additional measurements of maximum flow at small lung volume or transit time indices to follow change in this age group. In contrast to the established prognostic significance of a reduced FEV_1, the long-term significance of changes in these other tests of course remains unknown.

RATE OF DECLINE IN FEV_1 IN ESTABLISHED DISEASE

Several longitudinal studies of patients with COAD have shown very similar mean rates of decline in FEV_1 in the range 60-75 ml/yr (Burrows et al., 1987). This is faster than in the generality of smokers but not dramatically so (Table I), and implies a cumulative excess loss of FEV_1 of perhaps 1.5 or 2.0 l over up to 50 years of smoking. Factors which may increase this loss include an earlier start to decline in FEV_1 as a young adult and a tendency not to achieve quite such large values of FEV_1 if smoking is started before lung growth is completed as a young adult. When studying relatively advanced disease, there are confounding effects which tend to reduce mean rates of decline in FEV_1. Thus the most rapidly declining individuals die and are lost from long-term follow-up. In contrast, individuals with advanced disease and very low FEV_1 can survive for 10 years or more (even with continued smoking) yet such individuals must have had accelerated decline in FEV_1 at some earlier period. Such individuals with 'burnt-out' disease will tend to be over-represented in follow-up studies.

Many published surveys also treat COAD as a homogenous disease that can be effectively separated from asthma. Some doubt is cast on this by a recent analysis of the characteristics and prognosis of individuals found to have an FEV_1 of less than 65 % predicted in a community survey in Tucson (Burrows et al., 1987). When individuals with a reported diagnosis of asthma, who also were either non-smokers and/or had positive allergy skin tests, were separated from those with classic COAD (who were all non-atopic smokers or ex-smokers), large differences in 10 year survival were found. Survival of the COAD group was no better than that of patients studied in Chicago 20 years earlier. Average rates of decline in FEV_1 were 5 ml per year in the asthma group and 70 ml per year in the COAD group. But these two polar groups only comprised 72 of the 117 identified individuals. The remaining 45 subjects were predominantly men, had similar mean age and FEV_1 to the other two groups at enrolment and similar smoking histories to individuals in the classic COAD group. But they differed from the group with classic COAD in showing more asthmatic features such as positive allergy skin tests, increased blood eosinophils, raised serum IgE and wheezing. This group had annual rates of decline in FEV_1 and survival intermediate between the groups classed as asthma and COAD presumably because their obstruction can be partially reversed by treatment. These results indicate that the attempt to divide individuals with persistent airways obstruction simply into those with asthma and COAD is an over-simplification and confirm the persistent view of Dutch workers that there are subgroups of patients with differing rates of decline in lung function, differing response to treatment and differing prognosis (Postma et al., 1986). In conducting trials of treatment of COAD it may be necessary therefore to concentrate on 'classic' patients without any asthmatic features.

DISCUSSION

Stockley. I think the apparent discrepancy between cessation of smoking and changes in small airways inflammation but no effect in FEV_1, is confounded by problems of definition. Firstly, smoking habits are not similar and the number consumed is not equivalent to the amount of smoke inhaled. Secondly, the FEV_1 is predominantly a measure of large airways function whereas Dr. Hogg has been discussing the inflammation of small airways. There may be ways of measuring airways inflammation such as radioaerosol uptake by the circulation that will change when smoking is stopped.

Pride. Of course, there is a large number of degrees of freedom between reported smoking history and 'dose' of any individual smoke component, so I do not think the prospects for setting the first point are even going to be good!

On the second point I would certainly <u>not</u> regard the FEV_1 as a test of large airways function except in normal lungs. But Dr. Hogg could have more direct information on this.

Hogg. The discrepancy between the data showing improved function on stopping smoking and our factors to measure a change in airways pathology could mean that we measured the wrong thing. For example exudate on to the airways surface could narrow airways and decrease function and could clear up quickly on stopping smoking. We could not measure this with our techniques.

Bleecker.   Dr. Pride, you discussed Burrow's data that was recently published in NEJM.

1) In the asthmatic group I, the decline in FEV_1 was shown to be less severe. However, these subjects had significant and often severe airflow obstruction. Would this mean that during their lifetime there was a period of rapid decline in FEV_1?

2) Do you think the group II subjects with accelerated decline in FEV_1 have both asthmatic or host inflammatory factors combined with exposure to cigarette smoke – both factors causing airway disease?

Pride. 1) I agree – a low FEV_1 implies accelerated decline in the past except in the rare instance where normal airway function has never developed.

2) Rephrasing your question. Group II subjects, do they refute to the Dutch hypothesis by showing the combination of smoking and asthma is not worse than group I results. I know Dr. Burrows is very emphatic that his results should <u>not</u> be interpreted that way as the smoking and asthmatic features in that group were not necessarily coincident in individual patients!

REFERENCES

Bande, J., Clement, J., and Van de Woestijne, K.P. (1980) Am. Rev. Respir. Dis. 122: 781-790.

Beaty, T.H., Menkes, H.A., Cohen, B.H., and Newill, C.A. (1984) Am. Rev. Respir. Dis. 129: 660-667.

Burrows, B., Bloom, J.W., Traver, G.A., and Cline, M.G. (1987) New Engl. J. Med. 317: 1309- 1314.

Burrows, B., Knudson, R.J., Camilli, A.E., Lyle, S.K., and Lebowitz, M.D. (1987) Am. Rev. Respir. Dis. 135: 788-793.

Burrows, B., Lebowitz, M.D., Camilli, A.E., and Knudson, R.J. (1986) Am. Rev. Respir. Dis. 133: 974-980.

Camilli, A.E., Burrows, B. Knudson, R.J., Lyle S.K., and Lebowitz, M.D. (1987) Am. Rev. Respir. Dis. 135: 794-799.

Dockery, D.W., Speizer, F.E., Ferris, B.G. Jr., Ware, J.H., Louis, T.A., and Spiro, A. III. (1988) Am. Rev. Respir. Dis. 137: 286-292.

Fletcher, C., and Peto, R. (1977) Br. Med. J. 1: 1645-1648.

Fletcher, C.M., Peto, R., Tinker, C.M., and Speizer, F.E. (1976) Oxford: Oxford University Press.

Huhti, E., and Ikkala, J. (1980) Eur. J. Respir. Dis. 61: 33-45.

Kauffmann, F., Drouet, D., Lellouch, J., and Brille, D. (1979) International Journal of Epidemiology. 8: 201-212.

Osmanliev, D.P., Davies, E.E., Joyce, H., and Pride, N.B. (1988) Eur. Respir. J. 1: 41S.

Peat, J.K., Woolcock, A.J., and Cullen, K. (1989) Thorax, in press.

Peto R., Speizer, F.E., Cochrane, A.L., Moore, F., Fletcher, C.M., Tinker, C.M., Higgins, I.T.T., Gray, R.G., Richards, S.M., Gilliland, J., and Norman-Smith, B. (1983) Am. Rev. Respir. Dis. 128: 491-500.

Postma, D.S., De Vries, K., Köeter, G.H., and Sluiter, H.J. (1986) Am. Rev. Respir. Dis. 134: 276-280.

Pride, N.B. (1985) Ann. Acad. Med. Singapore. 14: 496-502.

3) THE ROLE OF MEASUREMENTS OF AIRWAY RESPONSIVENESS

F.E. Hargreave, E. Helen Ramsdale, P.G. Gibson, Isabelle Pin,
J.A. Denburg, and J. Dolovich

Asthma Research Group, Department of Medicine, St. Joseph's
Hospital, and Departments of Medicine and Pediatrics, Health
Sciences Centre and McMaster University, Hamilton, Ontario,
Canada.

SUMMARY: In smokers with chronic airflow limitation (CAL), airway
hyperresponsiveness (AHR) to stimuli like methacholine, which act
directly on airway smooth muscle, are not specific for the
pathogenesis which is responsible for AHR to methacholine in
subjects with normal spirometry, nor predictive for a beneficial
effect of glucocorticosteroid (GCS) treatment. In contrast, AHR
to stimuli like hyperventilation, which act indirectly through
mediator release, may be specific for the pathogenesis of asthma
and predictive for a beneficial effect of GCS. The validation of
this possibility requires the demonstration that patients with
CAL and AHR to hyper-ventilation demonstrate improvement after
treatment with GCS (and have an increase in eosinophils and
metachromatic cells in the sputum or bronchoalveolar lavage
(BAL), like that seen in asthmatics uncomplicated by CAL).

INTRODUCTION

Chronic bronchitis and asthma are still defined by clinical
criteria. Asthma is defined by an abnormality of function as
variable narrowing of the airways, and this includes the presence
of AHR. Chronic bronchitis is defined by cough and sputum. Both
conditions, however, appear to be caused by inflammation of the

airways. The characteristics of the inflammation differ, the inflammation of asthma being characterized by an increase in eosinophils and metachromatic cells (probably mucosal mast cells) (Gibson et al., 1989a, 1989b).

Chronic bronchitis and asthma can be complicated by CAL which can also occur in emphysema unassociated with either condition. The objective of this presentation is to discuss the possibility that certain measurements of airway responsiveness can be used to identify a GCS-responsive subgroup of patients with bronchitis and CAL.

DEFINITION AND MEASUREMENT OF AIRWAY HYPERRESPONSIVENESS

Airway hyperresponsiveness is defined as an increase in the magnitude and ease of airway narrowing to a variety of nonallergic (nonsensitizing) stimuli (Woolcock et al., 1984; Hargreave et al., 1986; Sterk & Bel, 1989). The stimuli can be divided into two groups, those which are considered to act directly on airway smooth muscle, eg. methacholine (or histamine), and those considered to act indirectly through release of chemical mediators, eg. hyperventilation, propranolol and methoxamine (Pauwels et al., 1988). AHR to both groups of stimuli is usual in patients with current asthma. In contrast, there is a difference in the ability of the two groups of stimuli to cause airway narrowing in normal subjects. Methacholine can cause airway narrowing in normal subjects if the dose is high, although the maximal degree of narrowing is limited to a relatively mild degree. The regulation of the dose delivered for inhalation is therefore critical to accurately interpret results. However, hyperventilation, propranolol or methoxamine do not appear to cause airway narrowing in normal subjects which suggests that they may be more specific for the pathogenesis of asthma.

AIRWAY HYPERRESPONSIVENESS IN ASTHMA

Methacholine AHR is a sensitive and specific test for asthma when spirometry is normal and when asthma is defined physiologically as variable airflow limitation (Hargreave et al., 1985). The presence and severity of methacholine AHR correlates closely with the presence and severity of variable airflow limitation as indicated by an increase in the diurnal variation of PFR and by the minimal treatment required to control symptoms. The baseline FEV_1 is usually normal until there is a moderate to severe increase in methacholine responsiveness. The degree of methacholine AHR can also correlate with the degree of responsiveness to hyperventilation, although this has not been demonstrated in all studies.

The presence and severity of methacholine AHR also correlates closely with the presence of airway inflammation of a special type and with a beneficial effect of treatment with GCS. For example, in people with mild stable asthma and with normal spirometry the presence and severity of methacholine AHR can correlate with the presence and severity of increases in eosinophils and metachromatic cells (mast cells or basophils) in BAL (Kirby et al., 1987; Wardlaw et al., 1988). When such subjects are given anti-inflammatory treatment with GCS, methacholine AHR usually becomes less (Ryan et al., 1985; Kraan et al., 1988). Furthermore, there is a close association between the heightening of airway responsiveness and the development of airway inflammation. For example, airway responsiveness to methacholine can be heightened after exposure to allergens and this correlates closely with the occurrence of late asthmatic responses which are associated with the cellular phase of airway inflammation (O'Byrne et al., 1987). This heightening of airway responsiveness can also be prevented or reversed by GCS treatment.

AIRWAY HYPERRESPONSIVENESS IN BRONCHITIS WITH OR WITHOUT CHRONIC AIRFLOW LIMITATION

In smokers with CAL, however, methacholine AHR is no longer specific for the same pathogenesis as in people with normal spirometry; nor is it predictive for an effect of GCS. In fact, when CAL is present (indicated by an FEV_1/VC of <70 %) airway responsiveness to methacholine is usually increased and the degree of increase shows a linear relationship to the severity of airflow limitation (Ramsdale et al., 1984). This suggests that the methacholine AHR in these patients with CAL may be secondary to the airflow limitation. Furthermore, methacholine AHR in patients with CAL is not improved by GCS (Koëter et al., 1989), unlike methacholine AHR in asthmatics. Finally, the degree of methacholine AHR is less than that in asthmatics without CAL but with a similar degree of airflow limitation at the time of the measurement, and there is usually no airway narrowing stimulated by hyperventilation, propranolol or methoxamine (Ramsdale et al., 1985; Woolcock et al., 1986; Du Toit et al., 1986). These features suggest that additional factors than airway calibre are responsible for the AHR in asthma and that AHR to hyperventilation, methoxamine and propranolol are specific for the pathogenesis of asthma and can be used to identify it when CAL is present. AHR to nonsensitizing stimuli which act through mediator release may therefore identify a subgroup of patients with CAL who will benefit from treatment with GCS. This possibility requires investigation.

Acknowledgements: This work is supported by grants from the Medical Research Council of Canada. We thank Mrs. Laurie Whitely for typing the manuscript.

DISCUSSION

Arborelius. The reproducibility of the FEV_1-test is about ± 100 ml. Thus in subjects with FEV_1 = 1 L a substantial number would get a decrease of up to 20 % of initial value just by chance while a change of 800 ml when starting at FEV_1 = 4 L would be highly significant. This could be avoided by expressing the changes in % of the predicted normal value.

Hargreave. The tests are usually not performed when the FEV_1 is this low because of safety and difficulty with interpreting the results. I don't know how results expressed in the way you suggest compare with expression as a percentage of baseline or post saline values.

Pride. The convention of normalizing to baseline FEV_1 arose empirically and it is not difficult to predict that responsiveness could increase disproportionally when baseline function is severely reduced.

Bleecker. Does histamine challenge, a so called direct stimulus, produce responses similar to methacholine in chronic obstructive bronchitis?

Hargreave. There is controversy but the differences, if present, are small and not useful to separate chronic obstructive bronchitis from asthma.

Laitinen. All our results support prof Hargreave's result that there is no obvious difference between histamine or methacholine bronchial hyperresponsiveness.

Larsson. Could you comment on the value of reversibility testing in patients with chronic airway obstruction? Can such testing identify individuals with variable airway obstruction?

Hargreave. They can identify variable airflow obstruction but not necessarily whether the pathogenesis is the same as in classical asthma.

REFERENCES

Du Toit, J.I., Woolcock, A.J., Salome, C.M., Sundrum, R., and Black, J.L(1986) Am. Rev. Respir. Dis. <u>134</u>, 498-501.

Gibson, P.G., Dolovich, J., Denburg, J., Ramsdale, E.H., and Hargreave, F.E(1989a) Lancet <u>i</u>, 1346-1348.

Gibson, P.G., Girgis-Gabardo, A., Morris, M.M., Mattoli, S., Kay, J.M., Dolovich, J., Denburg, J., and Hargreave, F.E (1989b) Thorax <u>44</u>, (in press).

Hargreave, F.E., Sterk, P.J., Ramsdale, E.H., Dolovich, J., and Zamel, N(1985) Chest <u>87</u>, S202-S206.

Hargreave, F.E., Dolovich, J., O'Byrne, P.M., Ramsdale, E.H., and Daniel, E.E(1986) J. Allergy Clin. Immunol. <u>78</u>, 825-832.

Kirby, J.G., O'Byrne, P.M., and Hargreave, F.E (1987) Am. Rev. Respir. Dis <u>135</u>, 554-556.

Koëter, G.H., Renkema, T.E.J., Auffarth, B., van der Mark, Th.W., de Monchy, J.G.R., Postma, D.S., and Kauffman, H.F. (1989) In: Glucocorticoids and Mechanisms of Asthma. Clinical and Experimental Aspects, (F.E.Hargreave, J.C.Hogg, J.L. Malo and J.H.Toogood, Eds), Excerpta Medica, Amsterdam, pp.148-156.

Kraan, J., Koëter, G.H., van der Mark, Th.W., Boorsma, M., Kukler, J., Sluiter, H.J., and de Vries, K (1988) Am. Rev. Respir. Dis. <u>137</u>, 44-48.

O'Byrne, P.M., Dolovich, J., and Hargreave, F.E (1987) Am. Rev. Respir. Dis. <u>136</u>, 740-751.

Pauwels, R., Joos, G., and van der Straeten, M. (1988) Clin. Allergy <u>18</u>, 317-321.

Ramsdale, E.H., Morris, M.M., Roberts, R.S., and Hargreave, F.E. (1984) Thorax <u>39</u>, 912-918.

Ramsdale, E.H., Roberts, R.S., Morris, M.M., and Hargreave, F.E. (1985) Thorax <u>40</u>, 422-426.

Ryan, G., Latimer, K.M., Juniper, E.F., Roberts, R.S., and Hargreave, F.E. (1985) J. Allergy Clin. Immunol. <u>75</u>, 25-30.

Sterk, P.J., and Bell, E.H (1989) Eur. Respir. J. <u>2</u>, 267-274.

Wardlaw, .J., Dunnette, S., Gleich, G.J., Collins, J.V., and Kay, A.B. (1988) Am. Rev. Respir. Dis. <u>137</u>, 62-69.

Woolcock, A.J., Salome, C.M., and Yan, K. (1984) Am. Rev. Respir. Dis. <u>130</u>, 71-75.

Woolcock, A.J., Cheung, W., and Salome, C. (1986) Am. Rev. Respir. Dis. <u>133</u>, A177.

AAS 30:
Inflammatory Indices
in Chronic Bronchitis
© 1990 Birkhäuser Verlag Basel

4) EFFECTS OF CORTICOSTEROIDS IN "CHRONIC BRONCHITIS" AND "CHRONIC OBSTRUCTIVE AIRWAY DISEASE"

Dirkje S. Postma, Tineke E.J. Renkema, and G.H. Koëter

Department of Pulmonology, University Hospital, Oostersingel 59, 9713 EZ Groningen, The Netherlands

SUMMARY: In order to improve our knowledge concerning the supposedly beneficial effects of corticosteroids in patients with "chronic bronchitis" and "chronic obstructive airway disease" (COAD), it is necessary to define our patients carefully, so that every investigator can interpret the data adequately. Up to now, no definite conclusion can be drawn as to the profitable effect of corticosteroids in COAD. A combination of data from many studies on oral and inhaled corticosteroids strongly suggests that long-term studies in large groups of patients are essential if we wish to determine a potential treatment effect. In this way, a sub-group of patients who improve on corticosteroids may be found too. In addition to objective measurements, e.g. degree of airflow obstruction and airway hyperresponsiveness (AH), subjective data and information on the patient's quality of life and exacerbations should be included for evaluation.

INTRODUCTION

It has been shown that inhaled corticosteroids can progressively change airway hyperresponsiveness in asthma. However, the effects of corticosteroids in patients with chronic obstructive airway disease (COAD) are still uncertain. This could indicate that the characterization of patient groups may have an important part to play when it comes to estimating responses to corticosteroids. It seems, therefore, necessary to define the diseases featuring diffuse airflow obstruction: asthma, chronic bronchitis, and COAD.

ATS and other guidelines are not very helpful in this respect. They all show that pure forms of the diseases are exceptional by stating, for instance, that "asthma is characterized by increased airway hyperresponsiveness", and that "airway hyperresponsiveness may be present in COAD"; "many patients with COAD have excess sputum production". This is in accordance with clinical practice, where most of the patients are not easily categorized as belonging to one disease group. The question then arises whether we need a diagnostic label for the treatment of patients or for scientific work. As so much overlap exists between asthma, COAD, and chronic bronchitis, we may be better off without a label so as to prevent confusion over the individual interpretation of that label. It seems, however, of great importance to describe our patients well in all our reports. This may afford valuable insights into the type of patients that has been studied; it may support comparisons of data, and it may make the generalization of the data, extending their significance to other patients, possible. Hence, it is necessary to provide at least the most important characteristics of the patients, e.g. age, gender, smoking history, level of airflow obstruction and reversibility, degree of allergy, airway hyperresponsiveness, and complicating factors such as frequent bacterial infections and bronchiectasis. If every report were to provide these data, the joint accumulation of results will supply information as to whether corticosteroids are beneficial in patients with "chronic bronchitis" and "COAD".

Corticosteroids have been used in the treatment of asthma and COAD since 1950, when the first preparations of biosynthetically derived analogues of the adrenal cortical hormones became available. Today, some 40 years later, their role in the management of COAD is still a controversial issue, whereas their use in asthma is firmly established. Oral and inhaled corticosteroids exert a beneficial effect on the degree of

airflow obstruction and airway hyperresponsiveness (AH) in
asthma, both after short-term and longer treatment periods. With
regard to COAD, several reports of short-term effects on the
degree of airflow obstruction have been submitted. Literature on
the long-term effects of oral corticosteroids and the effects of
inhaled corticosteroids with regard to the level of airflow
obstruction is scarce. Reports on the modulation of AH are even
harder to find.

SHORT-TERM EFFECTS OF ORAL AND INHALED CORTICOSTEROIDS

Those initial conflicts regarding the short-term benefit of oral
prednisolone in COAD that arose in the 1950's and 60's may
largely have resulted from the fact that studies on case series,
observational cohort studies,or non-randomized studies were
presented. Many well-documented double-blind, randomized,
placebo-controlled studies have followed. This study design is
the most reliable way of evaluating therapy. Results from these
trials are, however, also conflicting. The interpretation of
studies on therapy are hampered by several problems, for instance
the matching of groups and study conditions, the size of groups,
the variability of the measured parameters, and poor characterization on the part of the patient groups. Some studies, therefore, use a cross-over design (Evans et al., 1974; Shim et al.,
1978; Mendella et al., 1982; O'Reilly et al., 1982; Stokes et
al., 1982; Lam et al., 1983; Mitchell et al., 1984; Strain et
al., 1985; Eliasson et al., 1986;) with a washout period in order
to ensure optimal matching of compared groups and study
conditions. They require patients to be in a stable condition at
baseline in order to diminish the known beneficial effects of
corticosteroids in an acute exacerbation. Random variation in
spirometry is often considerable in patients with severe airflow
obstruction, and this can be mistaken for a treatment response
(O'Reilly et al., 1982; Stokes et al., 1982). Therefore, a
placebo period should always be included for each patient, or, as

Stokes et al. (1982) suggested, a run-in observation period of at least 3 months in order to determine within-patient variability. Small patient groups may also be a problem, their size prevents them from being representative of the general population with COAD.

Short-term effect on the FEV$_1$ level: When the above mentioned considerations are (more or less) taken into account, a few studies still remain worthwhile for evaluation of the short-term effects (1-2 weeks) of oral corticosteroids in COAD. Table I presents the available data of these selected studies.

"Responders" were defined as having a more than 20 % increase of FEV$_1$ in the corticosteroid period over placebo (baseline) FEV$_1$. It might have been very useful to provide another definition, e.g. the increase of FEV$_1$ as percentage of the predicted FEV$_1$, but more data were not available from the articles. It is clear that all studies show some responders except from one study (Evans et al., 1974), where a low dose of corticosteroids (5 mg) was given for 7 days. The lack of effect is most probably not due to duration of treatment, as it has been shown that most patients achieve their maximal response within 8 days. However, the dosage of 5 mg in this study is far lower than the 40 mg used for establishment of the maximum response. Thus, as for inhaled corticosteroids in asthma, there may exist not only a time-effect but also a dose-effect relationship.

The influence of patient characteristics on the response to corticosteroids: It has been suggested (Eliasson et al., 1986) that the percentage of patients who benefit from corticosteroid therapy as a result of an increase in their FEV$_1$, is over-estimated due to biased selection. Most studies evaluate patients with severe obstruction. Eliasson et al. (1986) found a signifi-cant negative correlation between the proportion of cortico-steroid responders and the mean FEV$_1$ level in 6 studies. Responders were differently defined in these studies. However, as responses have always been defined as percentage increases above

Table I. Baseline data and corticosteroid response of selected studies

	1	2	3	4	5	6	7	8	9	10
No of patients	16	10	16	46	43	10	24	13	31	57
dose of steroids, mg/day	40	5	40	32	40	30	30	32	30	40
Duration *, days	14	7	14	14	14	14	7	14	14	8
Responders*, %	12	0	43	17	35	30	33	8	13	7
, no	2	0	7	8	15	3	8	1	4	4
age , yrs	60	62	63	74	60	61	–	63	63	56
male , %	100	100	96	85	76	100	83	92	64	100
history of allergy**	no	no	no	yes	yes	–	no	no	no	no
eosinophil excess	yes	no	yes	yes	yes	–	yes	no	–	no
FEV_1 , L	1.24	1.11	0.85	1.03	1.02	0.81	0.74	1.16	0.84	1.98
FEV_1, %pred, %	35	–	33	37	37	–	27	–	–	63
FVC , L	2.74	2.28	1.92	–	2.22	2.56	–	2.43	2.15	–
FEV_1/FVC , %	45	49	45	–	44	–	–	48	–	45
FEV_1 , ml	120	90	85	156	160	162	177	70	–	200
FEV_1, %in , %	12	13	10	15	15	21	27	6	–	12
Sputum production, %	100	100	61	–	82	80	100	–	–	63

Effect prednisolone above placebo on

	1	2	3	4	5	6	7	8	9	10
FEV_1 , ml	112	–3	18	110	150	34	15	100	82	–50
FVC , ml	27	–2	22	–	200	159	–	0	119	–
PEFR , l/min	–	–	44	–	23	–	–	–	9	–
Complaints ,	no	–	yes	–	yes	yes	yes	4	–	yes
12 MD , m	–	–	47	–	52	38	–	–	–	–

1) Eliasson; 2) Evans; 3) Lam; 4) Mendella; 5) Mitchell; 6) O'Reilly; 7) Shim; 8) Strain; 9) Stokes; 10) Renkema (first authors, see REFERENCES)
– data not available
* > 20 % increase in FEV_1 on prednisolone above placebo
** personal or family history of atopy
 FEV_1: increase in FEV_1 after inhaled beta-agonist
12MD: 12 min walking distance

baseline, more responders can be expected in the region of a low baseline FEV_1: an increase of 200 ml above a baseline FEV_1 of 800 ml is 25 %, above 1500 ml it is 13 %. Hence, we took a closer look at the available data. Figure 1 shows that there is, as was to be expected, a significant (though not as high as stated in Eliasson et al., 1986) negative correlation (r=0.76, p<0.05) between the percentage of responders in each of the 9 studies and their respective mean baseline FEV_1. This significant negative correlation between the percentage of responders and baseline absolute FEV_1 persisted in the 5 studies in which the predicted FEV_1 percentage values were provided too (r=0,66, p<0.05). However, when the percentage of responders was correlated with the predicted FEV_1 percentage in the latter 5 studies, the significant correlation disappeared (r=0.44, p<0.05). Moreover, no significant correlation existed between baseline FEV_1 (Eliasson et al., 1986) and the absolute increase of FEV_1 (r=0.48, p<0.05). Thus, a response may occur irrespective of baseline FEV_1.

We have evaluated a group of patients with COAD and mild to moderate airflow obstruction (FEV_1>1.25 l, FEV_1%VC<60 %, RV%pred >120 %, PC_{20} histamine 5.37 [30 sec. tidal breathing method], no allergy according to skin test, eosinophils <250 /mm^3, and IgE <100 IU). The clinical characteristics are presented in Table I (study number 10). No patients used any inhaled or oral corticosteroids during three months before each investigation. Investigations took place after 8 days of placebo and after 8 days of 40 mg/day prednisolone orally, in a randomized order. The mean FEV_1 value was 1.98 l. In this patient population there were only 4 responders. Moreover, the mean FEV_1 even decreased on prednisolone. Thus, responders and non-responders seem to exist with FEV_1 values on a wide scale. This finding suggests that other factors than baseline FEV_1 must predict corticosteroid response in groups and in individual patients. A higher eosinophil count has been mentioned as such a factor (Shim et al., 1978; Eliasson et al., 1986), although others have been unable to find this (Evans et al., 1974; Mendella et al., 1982; Lam et al., 1983; Mitchell et al., 1984). Taken altogether, it appears that those studies that show an excess of eosinophils in the peripheral blood (Evans et al., 1974; Shim et al., 1978; Mendella et al., 1982; Lam et al., 1983; Eliasson et al., 1986) have a higher proportion of responders (mean 28 %) on corticosteroids than studies with low eosinophil counts (mean 5 %; Evans et al., 1974; Strain et al., 1985).

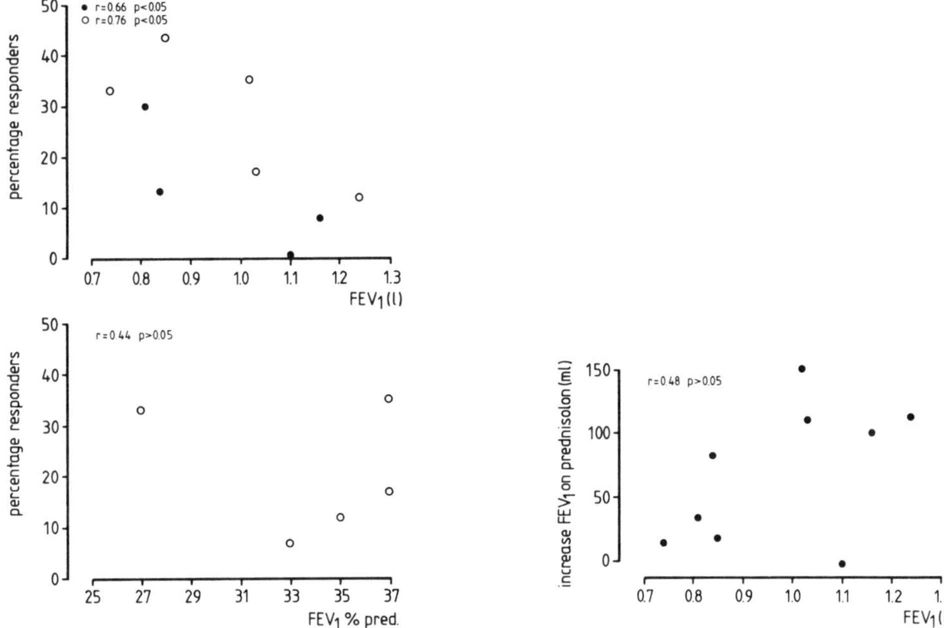

Figure 1. __Above left__: relation between percentage corticosteroid responders (%) and absolute baseline FEV_1 in 9 studies. O: studies in which FEV_1%pred values were not provided (n=4); O: studies in which FEV_1%pred values were provided (n=5)

__Below left__: relation between percentage corticosteroid responders (%) and baseline FEV_1 expressed as a percentage of the predicted value (%).

__Right__: relation between absolute increase of FEV_1 on prednisolone (ml) and absolute baseline FEV_1

FEV_1:   forced expiratory volume in one second.
FEV_1%pred: FEV_1 expressed as a percentage of the predicted value.
Responders: defined as having a more than 20 % increase of FEV_1 on corticosteroid treatment over placebo (baseline) FEV_1

The latter 2 studies also showed the lowest reversibility on a beta-adrenergic drug. As Mendella et al. (1982) suggested that higher reversibility on a beta-adrenergic drug precluded a greater response to corticosteroids, this might be important. Other studies did not support this observation. We could not find an overall significant correlation between reversibility and corticosteroid responsiveness in these 9 studies (both absolute and as percentages above baseline). Further studies involving a greater number of patients, with sufficient variation in FEV_1 may have to elucidate whether eosinophils (or, of equal or greater importance: neutrophils?) and/or the degree of reversibility influence the outcome with regard to the short-term effects of oral corticosteroids.

Today, it is not known which patients gain benefit from oral corticosteroids. It is not even at all clear whether the effects of the high doses of corticosteroids in the above-mentioned studies will be maintained when the doses are tapered off to clinically acceptable doses. Only a small percentage of the responders in two studies (Mendella et al., 1982; Shim & Williams, 1985) could maintain their response on (low doses of) inhaled corticosteroids. However, a single-blind, placebo-controlled, cross-over study of Harding & Freedman (1978), without washout periods, suggests that 4 responders (22 % of their population) responded as well to 10 days of treatment with supervised steroid aerosol (800 μg betamethasone valerate) as to 30 mg of prednisolone. We have investigated 24 non-allergic, smoking patients with COAD (mean age 57 years, mean FEV_1%pred 53 %, range 32–74 %, geometric mean PC_{20} histamine 1.07 mg/ml). They were treated in a randomized, double-blind fashion with either placebo or 1.6 mg/day budesonide after a 2-week placebo period. The patients on budesonide improved their FEV_1 by 150 ml, but the difference was just below significance. In patients on placebo, FEV_1 decreased by 100 ml. A lack of significant effect might be due to the duration of the therapy. One of the flaws in all studies up to now is that the effects of long-term trials are not known. It may well be that the beneficial effects of corticosteroids consist in the prevention of acute exacerbations, a reduction of the need for emergency-room visits, and an improvement in the patient's quality of life. This approach, however, needs a large population for a potential treatment effect to be determined.

Effect on airway hyperresponsiveness: When airway hyper-responsiveness is diminished, acute attacks of breathlessness may be prevented. The diminishment of AH seems to be important in COAD, as the severity of AH has been shown to be related to the decline in FEV_1 over time: a higher degree of AH was related to a steeper fall in FEV_1 (Postma et al., 1986). Corticosteroids are known to reduce the degree of AH in patients with asthma. However, the few results pertaining to COAD are not promising. In the above-mentioned study of 57 patients with COAD (no. 10 in Table I), we evaluated the effect of 40 mg prednisolone on AH after 4 days. Twenty-five smokers (S) and 32 ex-smokers (ES) were investigated. Mean FEV_1 (S 61.5, ES 62.4 % predicted) and geometric mean PC_{20} histamine (S 4.72, ES 5.69 mg/ml) were not significantly different between S and ES on placebo. FEV_1 did not change significantly on prednisolone (S 59.6, ES 61.4%pred.) However, the PC_{20} histamine on prednisolone was significantly lower (almost one doubling dose) in smokers (geometric mean 3.78) than in ex-smokers (geometric mean 6.52 mg/ml). Results show that short-term oral cortico-steroids do not decrease AH in COAD. They could even lead to AH deterioration in smokers, possibly as a result of the fact that the deleterious effect of smoking continues, whereas the anti-inflammatory corticosteroids dampen the defence. This finding is supported by results obtained from the already mentioned 24 smokers with COAD: on placebo, the mean increase in PC_{20} after 8 weeks was 1.2 mg/ml, whereas the decrease in PC_{20} after 8 weeks of budesonide was 1.5 mg/ml. Pride et al. (1987) also mentioned that 3 months of 1200 μg budesonide did not influence AH or only did so to a small extent, and effects were not found in all subjects. Here, again, more comprehensive studies of longer duration are necessary in order to elucidate whether corticosteroids actually suppress AH in COAD, or perhaps in a sub-group of this patient category.

LONG-TERM EFFECTS OF CORTICOSTEROIDS

There are as yet no data on long-term, double-blind, placebo-controlled intervention studies with corticosteroids. In an open study, Deschepper (1974) showed that 3.5 to 12.5 months of treatment with injections of 40 mg methylprednisolone acetate every eight to fourteen days resulted in an improvement in peak flow in one out of 5 patients with COAD of whom data before and after treatment were available. The clinical result was considered to be fair or good in 7, and unsatisfactory in 4 patients. Results were better in patients who were also considered to have asthma (13 good or fair, 2 unsatisfactory). Two other studies (Postma et al., 1985, 1988), both of a retrospective nature, show a beneficial effect of cortico-steroids. It was observed in these studies that patients did not have a uniform pattern of FEV_1 at follow-up. In some patients, FEV_1 remained stable; in others there was a linear fall, or an increase followed by a decrease, and a fourth group showed a decrease followed by an increase. The groups were comparable with regard to age, sex, smoking habits, FEV_1, reversibility and AH. Therapy in the form of anticholinergics, theophylline, and betamimetics was virtually the same in all groups. A striking association existed between the pattern of change in FEV_1 and intake and dosage of oral prednisolone. Below a dosage of 10 mg prednisolone (e.g. 7.5 or 5 mg), FEV_1 declined continuously. When 10 mg or more prednisolone was given, FEV_1 remained stable or even improved. A strong correlation existed between the institution or increase of oral corticosteroids to 10 mg or more per day and an increase in FEV_1. Conversely, both studies showed that a reduction below 10 mg or cessation of prednisolone resulted in a decline in FEV_1.

These two studies contain results from 129 patients with

severe airflow obstruction (FEV_1%pred 25 %, FEV_1%VC 27 %) and 139 with moderately severe airflow obstruction (FEV_1%pred 63 %, FEV_1%VC 48 %). They were of a retrospective character, and had a long follow-up (14-20 yrs), but any interpretation of the data should be carried out carefully. Nevertheless, 53 patients can be considered as being their own controls, as corticosteroids were instituted or withheld during follow-up in these patients.

It took between 6 months and 2 years before the effects of corticosteroids on FEV_1 could be observed in these studies. This is in striking contrast to patients with asthma, where effects with even lower doses of corticosteroids often show within a few weeks. It indicates, however, that when new prospective studies are to be started, a long follow-up may be necessary to determine a response to corticosteroids. In the light of current knowledge regarding the side effects of corticosteroids, it is certainly not warranted to start all patients with COAD on 10 mg of oral prednisolone. It seems worthwhile to investigate whether inhaled steroids, or a combination of inhaled and oral corticosteroids, have the same beneficial effect.

Where the effect of corticosteroids on the long-term course of FEV_1 is concerned, there is uncertainty regarding the mechanisms involved. Patient selection might have influenced the results. It has been suggested that corticosteroids provide a better response in patients with higher reversibility (Mendella et al., 1982), eosinophilia and atopy (Eliasson et al., 1986). However, patients with atopy and eosinophilia were carefully excluded (Postma et al., 1988), and each of the four groups with a specific course on FEV_1 included 25 % patients with a less than 20 % increase of FEV_1 on a bronchodilator. We have suggested that the results may stem from a modulating effect of corticosteroids on AH. This may be caused by a dampening of the inflammatory processes which are thought to be the underlying mechanism of AH.

Glucocorticosteroids are known to suppress acute and chronic inflammation, irrespective of cause, by inhibiting virtually every step in the inflammatory process, for instance by means of a redistribution of leukocytes in various body pools, by influencing chemotactic and vasoactive substances and by reducing the leakage of fluids and cells into inflammatory loci by constricting the microvasculature.

Polymorphonuclear leukocytes seem to be the important cells with regard to inflammatory processes in COAD (with or without sputum production), as opposed to eosinophils in asthma. These former cells contain proteolytic enzymes which produce mucus gland hyperplasia, reduce ciliary beat frequency, and damage ciliated epithelium (Stockley, 1988). Moreover, patients with COAD and sputum production are known to have significant losses of plasma proteins in their sputum, which are potentially harmful to e.g. the epithelium. All these effects may potentiate AH. Corticosteroids may stabilize lysosomal membranes and decrease protease release, and also inhibit the generation of toxic oxygen products. They may reduce the basal release of mucus and the response of bronchial explants to secretagogues in vitro, which is consistent with the clinical observation of their beneficial effect in bronchorrhea (Stockley, 1988).

However, short-term studies of corticosteroids in AH and COAD seem to refute the hypothesis that corticosteroids affect AH. As inflammatory processes in COAD involve other cells than in asthma, it is still possible that a different dose or duration of therapy is required. Also, we cannot disregard the possibility that the positive long-term effects may result from the corticosteroid effect on the proteinase-antiproteinase balance in favour of the inhibitors (Stockley, 1988).

Acknowledgement: Part of the studies in this article have been made possible by the "Netherlands Asthma Foundation".

DISCUSSION

Pride. Are you saying there is no relation between the short-term response (over the first 1-3 weeks) and the long-term response to oral corticosteroids?

Tineke Renkema.   Most short-term studies on the effects of corticosteroids in COAD show only a small percentage of steroid-responders. The two long-term studies that were performed in our department by Dr. Postma show that treatment with prednisolone (in a dose of 10 mg or more per day) may be effective in slowing down progression of disease in patients with COAD. However, it took 6-24 months before the effects of prednisolone treatment became visible. This suggests that response to corticosteroid treatment may be underestimated in short-term trials due to duration of the study, and that more responders might be found when studies of longer duration are performed.

Gibson.   When the underlying hypothesis considers airway inflammation as causing illness, and when patients are treated with an anti-inflammatory drug, it seems inappropriate to use a measure of air flow limitation as the outcome assessment. Would it be better to use a measure of airway inflammation as the outcome assessment?

Tineke Renkema.   I agree that inflammatory parameters should be included in studies investigating the effectiveness of corticosteroid treatment. I think, however, that the problem is that as yet we do not know which parameters are the most suitable and/or valuable in this respect.

Löfdahl.   We are approaching the fundamental question whether we like to study a broad patient material where COAD is part of it, or if we want to study a "pure" COAD group of patients. I think we should try to focus on "pure" COAD, to evaluate if gluco-corticosteroids have a therapeutic effect.

Tineke Renkema.   I totally agree. We know that glucocorticoids have a beneficial effect in "asthma". From short-term studies on the effects of glucocorticoids in COAD, we know that those patients likely respond to treatment often have signs of "asthma", like excess of eosinophils. What we do _not_ know is whether patients with "pure" COAD respond to treatment with GCS, and, if so, which patients are likely to respond, so I suggest we should concentrate on these patients with "pure" COAD.

Hargreave. I disagree with the exclusion of patients with chronic airflow limitation who have features consistent with asthma.

Persson. In your analysis of factors involved in the various courses of obstruction development you said that "broncho-dilators" had no influence. I think you need to treat xanthines, β-agonists and antimuscarinics as separate drug interventions because they have different effects, one of which may be broncho-dilation.

Tineke Renkema. I agree, but the number of patients was too small for this subanalysis.

Laitinen. There are some difficulties in measuring markers of inflammation in sputum after inhaled glucocorticoids, because this treatment may dramatically decrease the sputum production. What is the effect of inhaled glucocorticoid treatment on BAL fluid cell count?

Tineke Renkema. In our study on the short-term effects of oral prednisolone in COAD, we saw no effect of prednisolone treatment on total cell count of BAL fluid, nor on the number of cells per ml of BAL fluid. In the differentiation of BAL cells, predni-solone treatment induced a small but insignificant reduction of the percentage of neutrophils and a small, significant reduction in the percentage of eosinophils. Before treatment with prednisolone, however, thus on placebo, these percentages were not significantly different in COAD patients and matched healthy controls.

Laitinen. What is the need of short course oral corticosteroid trial in characterization of CB or COAD in patients?

Koëter. With a short course of corticosteroids "hidden asthmatics" can be identified. To find "responders" in older patients with an obstructive lung disease more prolonged courses are needed.

Widdicombe. The Ciba Foundation of chronic bronchitis emphasizes maintained production of sputum as the primary diagnostic feature of the disease. The recent ATS definition omits sputum production. Do you think assessment of volume of sputum production (as distinct from its chemical and cellular analysis) has any value in differential diagnosis of chronic bronchitis and other obstructive airways diseases?

Koëter. Sputum production can be considered as the consequences of an obstructive lung disease (asthma, COAD). To assess what is in the sputum is very important. I would guess that eosinophils, which are quite often seen in patients with COAD would predict a good glucocorticoid response.

Gibson. Sputum is useful in the assessment of patients. It is non-invasive and can be used to document the characteristics of the inflammatory cell infiltrate.

Koëter. I agree that investigating sputum will provide a good indication of inflammatory processes in the airways. However, not all patients produce sputum and I am not sure whether an assessment of sputum is well reproducible.

Stockley. I would like to make two brief comments. Firstly, just assessing sputum volume may prove useful in assessing response to steroid therapy. I have been collaborating in a study of inhaled steroids and we wished to examine biochemical factors in sputum. As the study progressed we lost some patients as their sputum production ceased. Secondly, if the patient produces sputum, lung lavage data appears from our own studies to be almost identical.

Larsson. Is eosinophilia a clinical characteristic of importance to distinguish asthma from COAD?

Koëter. Eosinophils can be observed both in asthmatics and in patients with COAD. Eosinophils certainly do not separate asthma from other lung diseases. The presence of eosinophils in the airways will not always lead to bronchial hyperresponsiveness.

Hogg. Does sputum reflect central airways or peripheral airways or both?

Koëter. In fact I don't know. I would expect that sputum reflects mainly the events going on in the larger airways.

Arborelius. Normal subjects improve FEV_1 by 100 ml ±SD (50 ml) after bronchodilating compound. An abnormal increase would thus be >200 ml and >250 ml and may only be seen in asthmatics. At least we have to define what increase indicates "reversibility" in an asthmatics.

Koëter. Reversibility can be expressed as: 1) absolute increase in FEV_1, 2) percentage increase from initial FEV_1, 3) increase expressed in % of predicted FEV_1, and 4) FEV_1, % (predicted - initial). I prefer an expression bringing in predicted FEV_1.

Arborelius. Pride asked whether breathlessness can be measured. Breathlessness cannot be measured since it is a subjective feeling of the patient. Very often lung function can decrease very much in a patient before they get short of breath because they adapt to their condition. However, several studies have shown that decreases in peak flow measurements in the morning predict subjective breathlessness in a patient so that therapy can counteract breathlessness or serious clinical deterioration of asthma.

REFERENCES

Deschepper, P. (1974) Acta Tub. et Pneum. Belgica 2, 243-248.

Eliasson, O., Hoffman, J., Trueb, D., Frederick, D., and McCormick, R. (1986) Chest. 4, 484-490.

Evans, JA., Morrison, IM., and Saunders, KB. (1974) Thorax 29, 401-406.

Harding, SM., and Freedman, S. (1978) Thorax 33, 214-218.

Lam, WK., So, SY., Yu, DYC. (1983) Br. J. Dis. Chest. 77, 189-198.

Mendella, LA., Manfreda, J., Warren, CPW., Anthonisen, NR. (1982) Annals of Internal Medicine 96, 17-21.

Mitchell, DM., Gildeh, P., Rehahn, M., Dimond, AH., and Collins, JV. (1984) Lancet ii, 193-195.

O'Reilly, JF., Shaylor, JM., Fromings, KM., and Harrison, BDW. (1982) Br. J. Dis. Chest 76, 374-382.

Postma, DS., De Vries, K., Koëter, GH., and Sluiter, HJ. (1986) Am. Rev. Respir. Dis. 134, 276-280.

Postma, DS., Peters, I., Steenhuis, EJ., and Sluiter, HJ. (1988) Eur. Respir. J. 1, 22-26.

Postma DS., Steenhuis EJ., Weele LTh van der., and Sluiter, HJ. (1985) Eur. J. Respir. Dis. 67, 56-64.

Pride, NB., Taylor, RG., Lim, TK., Joyce, H., and Watson, A. (1987) Bull. Eur. Physiopathol. Respir. 23, 369-375.

Renkema, TEJ., Postma, DS., and Sluiter, HJ. (1988) Am. Rev. Respir. Dis. 137 (4., part 2), 242.

Shim, C., Stover, DE., Williams Jr., MH. (1978) J. Allergy Clin. Immunol. 62, 363-367.

Shim, CS., and Williams Jr., MH. (1985) Am. J. Med. 78, 655-658.

Stockley, RA. (1988) Clinics in Chest Medicine 9, 643-656.

Stokes, TC., O'Reilly, JF., Shaylor, JM., and Harrison, BDW. (1982) Lancet ii, 345-348.

Strain, DS., Kinasewitz, GT., Franco, DP., and George, RB. (1985) Chest 88, 718-721.

5) EPIDEMIOLOGY OF OBSTRUCTION, EXACERBATIONS AND HYPER-REACTIVITY. EFFECTS OF GLUCOCORTICOSTEROIDS AND OTHER ANTI-INFLAMMATORY TREATMENT

N.B. Pride

Department of Medicine, Royal Postgraduate Medical School
LONDON, W12 ONN, United Kingdom

SUMMARY: Validated and standardized questions are available for self-reporting of exacerbations of symptoms due to broncho-pulmonary infections but not for non-infective exacerbations. The presence of non-specific bronchial hyperresponsiveness may help to identify smokers with a high risk of rapid decline in lung function, but change in bronchial responsiveness with treatment probably cannot be used to predict subsequent long-term progression in FEV_1. In non-asthmatic individuals three months' treatment with glucocorticosteroids has not improved FEV_1 nor reduced bronchial responsiveness; the effects of glucocortico-steroids on bronchial secretions and infections and long-term decline in FEV_1 are largely unknown.

INTRODUCTION

The major symptoms of patients with chronic obstructive airway disease (COAD) can be broadly divided into those associated with the airway narrowing - dyspnoea, wheezing - and those associated with chronic expectoration and the increased tendency to broncho-pulmonary infections. The studies of Fletcher et al. (1977), which distinguish between the obstructive and hypersecretory components of COAD, have resulted in greater emphasis being placed in recent years on the obstructive component because of its established prognostic importance.

In attempting to modify the insidious course of chronic airways obstruction by treatment, three rather different types of favourable responses can be postulated:-
1)   a sustained improvement in symptoms in the chronic stable state - this could be due to an improvement in FEV_1 and/or to a reduction in chronic cough and expectoration
2)   a reduction in the frequency or length of exacerbations of symptoms
3)   a slowing of the progressive decline in FEV_1 after the start of treatment.

Clearly the third type of response requires considerable effort to prove or disprove and there are no a priori grounds for predicting that the absence of an improvement in the first two types of response predicts that there will be no long-term benefit. This had led to some of the current interest in bronchial hyper-responsiveness (BHR) in chronic airways obstruction. Is BHR a predictor of subsequent accelerated decline in FEV_1? If so, does attenuation of BHR provide an early indication of slowing of long-term decline in FEV_1? Attenuation of BHR might be associated also with reduction in non-infective exacerbations of breathlessness, some of which might be related to environmental factors such as air pollution and cold weather.

In this paper, I will briefly discuss the prevalence of obstruction and of exacerbations of symptoms and of the role of BHR as an indicator of the decline in FEV_1. Finally, I will review the available data on the effects of glucocorticosteroid and other anti-inflammatory treatment.

PREVALENCE OF AIRWAYS OBSTRUCTION

There is much more information on the prevalence of respiratory symptoms than of airways obstruction in the community. In part, this is because of the difficulty in defining airways obstruction. The simplest solution is to define a boundary below which airways obstruction is present, as in the widely quoted study of Higgins et al. (1982) who used FEV_1 <65 % predicted (provided FEV_1/FVC was also <80 %). Using this criterion, 10-15 % of men and about 5 % of women between 45 and 64 years had airways obstruction. Inevitably most of these subjects will have values only a little below the chosen boundary. Another popular criterion is FEV_1/FVC below 60 % (see review in Surgeon General's 1984 report on 'The Health Consequences of Smoking'). A few studies provide more detailed information on the distribution of values in at-risk groups - such as smokers or various occupational groups - as compared with a healthy non-smoking reference population (Burrows et al., 1977; Dockery et al., 1988).

RECORDING EXACERBATION OF SYMPTOMS

The British Medical Research Council Questionnaire on respiratory symptoms contains standard questions for documenting the reported occurrence of exacerbations of infections, and this has been the basis for most subsequent studies of exacerbations (e.g. Anthonisen et al., 1987). As far as I know, no comparable questions have been developed for documenting non-infective exacerbations not associated with increased volume and purulence of sputum. In the winter trials of antibiotics in the nineteen-sixties, there was a reduction in the number of infective exacerbations in the minority of individuals who had very frequent exacerbations. There was also some shortening of time off work per exacerbation. Three studies in the nineteen-eighties have examined the effects of treatment with oral N-acetylcysteine on the number and length of exacerbations of symptoms (Boman et al., 1983; British Thoracic Society Research Committee, 1985; Multicenter Study Group, 1980) [Table I]. These studies have retained definitions of exacerbations similar to those used in the nineteen-sixties. There are considerable problems with self-reporting of infections - especially at frequent intervals - and over the years, the clinical impression is that the exacerbations are milder and antibiotic treatment is started earlier. In the N-acetyl cysteine trials also, the number of reported exacerbations varied considerably between individuals and obviously there is the greatest potential for improvement in the minority of subjects who report the largest number of exacerbations when not on active treatment. This is the equivalent of the subject with rapid decline in FEV_1.

Table I. Exacerbation of infection rate per winter in multicentre trials of oral N-acetylcysteine treatment.

	No. of subjects	Mean age (yrs)	FEV_1 % pred	Mean exacerbation rate/winter PLACEBO	ACETYL-CYSTEINE
Italian multi-centre group (1980)	495	--	>40 %	2.0	0.8
Swedish Society for Pulmonary Diseases (1983)	203	52	mean 80 %	1.7	1.2
British Thoracic Society (1985)	181	63	mean 30 %	2.6	2.1

I do not know if the individuals who report frequent exacerbations one winter, do so in subsequent winters nor whether they report less severe exacerbations than other individuals. Certainly, there are quite large differences in the rates of exacerbation while taking placebo between the three trials, although these may be related partly to differing severity of airway disease in the recruited subjects.

BRONCHIAL HYPERRESPONSIVENESS

The idea that bronchial hyperresponsiveness (BHR) was important in the pathogenesis of chronic airways obstruction was made first by Dutch workers in the early nineteen-sixties, who proposed that this hyperresponsiveness was genetically determined. Many studies since have confirmed that non-specific BHR - usually assessed as the response to inhaled histamine or methacholine - is found consistently in middle-aged male smokers with mild or moderate chronic airflow obstruction (Pride et al., 1987). The very large NHLBI study in North America, which also contains many women, confirms this association. Male smokers who have shown preceding, accelerated annual decline in forced expiratory volume in one second (FEV_1) show abnormal BHR to inhaled bronchoconstrictor or bronchodilator drugs. There is also an association between low baseline FEV_1 and an accelerated annual decline in FEV_1 ("horse-racing effect" or "tracking") at least in middle-aged male smokers. But none of these associations indicates whether BHR is important in pathogenesis or merely one of many unimportant consequences of smoking.

The two main theories about the origins of BHR in smokers - that it is specifically related to the presence of active inflammation of the airway wall or that it is merely a consequence of altered airway geometry - are difficult to distinguish because it is generally agreed that the altered geometry is itself the result of a current or past inflammatory process. Nevertheless, the differentiation is important because in one case the implication is that BHR is a pathogenetic factor in the development of obstruction, in the other merely a consequence of earlier damage.

There is abundant evidence of chronic inflammation, in expectorated sputum, in bronchoalveolar lavage fluid and in bronchial wall biopsies, in smokers studied in the stable state between exacerbations of bronchopulmonary infection. There is also a chronic elevation of neutrophil and total white blood cell (WBC) count in the peripheral blood. However, we have found no association between the presence of chronic expectoration or the increase in total WBC and BHR in smokers. A more direct way to assess the role of active inflammation in perpetuating BHR is to study the effects of anti-inflammatory interventions; even if BHR arose from a combination of active inflammation and established alteration in airway geometry, anti-inflammatory measures could reveal a reversible component to the BHR of smokers.

MEASURES TO REDUCE AIRWAY INFLAMMATION

Overall there is more extensive knowledge of the effect of stopping smoking than of drug treatment in patients with chronic airflow obstruction. For this reason it is useful to review the effects of stopping smoking before considering anti-inflammatory drugs.

Stopping smoking: Stopping smoking reduces chronic cough and expectoration and the frequency of exacerbation of broncho-pulmonary infections. In younger smokers there is usually some early improvement in airway function, but this is smaller or absent in older smokers. The effects of giving up smoking on BHR in non-asthmatic subjects are less clear. We have followed sixteen ex-smokers with BHR (who had already given up smoking when first found to have BHR) by repeating measurement of BHR and FEV_1 after an interval of four years (Pride et al., 1987). At the time of the first measurement, BHR at a given reduction in FEV_1 was slightly more intense in the ex-smokers than in a comparable group of continuing smokers. But after a further 4 years without smoking, BHR was quite unchanged and FEV_1 showed only the normal age-related decline over this period, probably due to loss of lung recoil, rather than to intrinsic airway narrowing. This result favours the importance of geometric factors rather than active airway inflammation. Of course we cannot exclude the possibility that ex-smokers with BHR are biased towards those with "endogenous", allergic BHR rather than to acquired, non-allergic, smoking-related BHR, and there was some evidence to support this. Nevertheless, some reduction in inflammation would surely be expected on stopping smoking. Better evidence would be provided by studying BHR before and after stopping smoking. Published studies are limited but fail to show any short-term attenuation of BHR; more definitive information should come from the large NHLBI study. In the few individuals we have followed, no attenuation of BHR has occurred.

Most importantly, despite the apparent lack of attenuation of BHR, many studies show that subsequent decline in FEV_1 in both younger and older smokers is slowed after giving up smoking to rates only slightly greater than in never-smokers.

Glucocorticosteroids: Assessment of the effects of glucocorticosteroids is complicated by the need to distinguish between asthmatic and non-asthmatic forms of chronic airways obstruction. While it is relatively easy to pick out classic asthmatic (or indeed classic non-asthmatic) individuals, many individuals have some asthmatic features as emphasized by the North American usage of chronic asthmatic bronchitis. This difficulty probably accounts for the short-term effects (2-3 weeks) of glucocorticosteroids on airway function in patients with chronic airway obstruction remaining uncertain, with some studies showing useful improvements in airway function (FEV_1 or PEF) at least in some individuals while others are completely negative (Stoller, 1989; Stoller et al, 1987). A similar controversy exists about the long-term effects of oral glucocorticosteroids on decline in FEV_1 (Postma et al., 1985).

In subjects with classic extrinsic asthma, inhaled corticosteroids have consistently produced a moderate attenuation of BHR to inhaled histamine over 2-3 months' treatment, possibly taking longer to reach a plateau of effect (Kraan et al., 1988). Recent studies also show attenuation of BHR in intrinsic asthma. I know of three studies of the effects of glucocorticoids on FEV_1 and bronchial responsiveness in smokers or patients with chronic bronchitis or chronic airways obstruction selected because of the absence of co-existing asthmatic features. None are fully published but all failed to show any improvement in baseline FEV_1 or attenuation of responsiveness.

Engel et al., (1989) carried out a 12 week trial of 800 μg inhaled budesonide per 24 hours in 8 smokers with chronic bronchitis with completely negative results. We have examined the effects of 12 weeks' treatment with 1200 μg budesonide inhaled per 24 hours in a double-blind cross-over trial in 14 middle-aged male smokers. The men were known to have had accelerated decline in FEV_1 over the preceding 12 years. We found no improvement in baseline FEV_1, no increase in the postbronchodilator FEV_1, no improvement in PEF measured at home over 2 weeks, and no attenuation of bronchial responsiveness to inhaled histamine. Six of the men completed 12 months of budesonide, and their progress was compared with six men who received no active treatment for the same period; no suggestion of a favourable response was obtained although, of course, the numbers were to small and the follow-up period too short to assess long-term change in FEV_1. The group from Groningen, who treated current smokers with developed airflow obstruction with 1600 μg budesonide per 24 hours, also failed to show any attenuation of BHR (Koëter et al., 1989). Hence, individuals chosen to be definitely non-asthmatic apparently show no improvement in FEV_1 or attenuation of BHR with three months' treatment with inhaled corticosteroids at doses, which consistently improve both these aspects in overtly asthmatic subjects. However, stopping smoking, which presumably has large anti-inflammatory effects, also does not consistently improve FEV_1 in the short-term or attenuate BHR, yet it is highly effective in attenuating future decline in FEV_1. So there can be no substitute for a prospective study of the effects of glucocorticosteroids on decline in FEV_1.

Other aspects of the effects of glucocorticosteroid treatment in chronic airways obstruction are largely unknown. Do they reduce the frequency or severity of non-infective exacerbations of breathlessness? In acute illness with fall in FEV_1, systemic glucocorticosteroids apparently accelerate recovery even in individuals who show no benefit in FEV_1 when elective trials are made in the chronic stable state (Albert et al., 1980). Conventionally, glucocorticosteroid treatment is associated with immune suppression and an increased propensity to infections, but physicians have not commented on this risk in patients treated with inhaled corticosteroids except for the increased risk of oro-pharyngeal candidiasis. Conceivably inhaled corticosteroids could reduce the exudative contribution to bronchial secretions which might have a similar effect to mucolytic drugs or stopping smoking; comment on this aspect is virtually confined to the beneficial effects of corticosteroids in gross "bronchorrhoea". A reduction in sputum volume or protein content might in turn reduce the frequency of broncho-pulmonary infections; presumably this is the reason mucolytic drugs or stopping smoking result in a reduced tendency to bronchial infection.

Other non-steroidal anti-inflammatory drugs: In normal subjects in whom BHR has been induced by breathing ozone, cyclo-oxygenase products have been increased in broncho-alveolar lavage fluid. Therefore, although cyclo-oxygenase inhibitors have not been useful in human asthma, it seemed possible that they might be more effective in smoking-induced airway inflammation. We have made two studies in middle-aged male smokers with mild airways obstruction. In the first, there was no change in BHR of FEV_1 one hours after a single 1,2 G dose of aspirin; in the second study, we obtained no change after treatment with another potent cyclo-oxygenase inhibitor, flurbiprofen. These studies, therefore, provide no evidence that cyclo-oxygenase products intensify BHR in smokers in the short-term; I know of no longer-term studies. There also appears to be little information on the effects of cromoglycate or nedocromil in smoking-related airways obstructions. This is more surprising now that it is recognized that these drugs may have prophylactic effects beyond those originally attributed to their effects on mast cells.

Antibiotics: Continuous prophylactic treatment with antibiotics slightly reduces the length of symptoms caused by infections, but studies in the nineteen-sixties failed to show slowing of decline in FEV_1 in "usual" patients with chronic airways obstruction (Pride, 1987). The antibiotic regimes used were often not those that would be chosen now, but this may not be critical in view of the difficulty there is in showing differing short-term effects of various current antibiotic regimes (Anthonisen et al., 1987).

Bronchodilators: Similarly with bronchodilator treatment, the only definite beneficial effect is the short-term improvement in FEV_1; The NHLBI study is currently examining whether long-term decline in FEV_1 is slowed by regular treatment with ipratropium bromide. We know that bronchodilators provide short-term attenuation of non-specific BHR so they might protect also against exacerbations of breathlessness induced by infective or non-infective causes. Beta-adrenergic agonists and theophyllines have some anti-inflammatory actions, which conceivably could have longer-term effects on mucosal inflammation and swelling.

Mucolytic Drugs: These reduce the number of exacerbations of infection (Table I) and possibly reduce the volume of sputum produced in the stable state (Multicenter Study Group, 1980). They also have anti-inflammatory effects, so again it is conceivable they could affect long-term decline in FEV_1.

CONCLUSION: It is evident from this brief review that whereas we are relatively familiar with the full range of effects of giving up smoking, we have only partial knowledge of the short- and long-term effects of drug treatment in smoking-related airways disease. Most of the drugs routinely used have effects additional to the primary effect for which they are prescribed, In all cases, the long-term effects are controversial if not completely unknown. It would be convenient if short-term attenuation of BHR by treatment was a useful predictor of the long-term effects of that treatment on decline in FEV_1, but this cannot be assumed to be the case. However, the presence of BHR probably does identify a high-risk, rapidly declining group of smokers, who could be selected for intervention studies.

DISCUSSION

Hogg. Did you establish the rate of decline in FEV_1 over the year of your budesonide study?

Pride. The men in our budesonide study had been followed for 12 years, and a group were fairly rapid decliners over this period. As for trying to obtain a control slope and then a slope during a placebo-controlled intervention, I expect this would make it easier to see any effect but it adds considerably to the length of the study.

Hogg. If only 20 % of the smokers get abnormalities, the 80 % who don't will introduce a lot of noise in the signal. Would it not be better to establish the rate of decline first and only introduce an intervention in the 20 % who are having a rapid decline?

Pride. This is undoubtedly true, but of course there is a trade-off into the increased duration of study needed if rapid decliners have to be identified by direct observation. We had hoped rapid decliners could be identified by age, number of cigarettes smoked, bronchial hyperresponsiveness but have had only limited success.

Skoogh. It shouldn't be necessary to follow subjects for a longer period of time to identify "rapid decliners". Just picking smokers with a reduced FEV_1 should give a high number of rapid decliners.

Pride. Yes, if they continue smoking.

Bleecker. There is an intervention study in the U.S. that is sponsored by the National Institute of Health - NHLBI - Lung Diseases Division. It consists of 10 study sites (throughout the U.S. and Canada) and a Data Center in Minnesota. The purpose of this study is to evaluate the effects of smoking cessation and pharmacologic therapy with an anticholinergic agent in the decline in FEV_1 over a five year period in 6000 subjects. Recruitment has been completed and the interventions are in progress.

Hogg. How long do you have to follow patients to be sure that they have a rapid decline?

Pride. Individual subjects take several years, but data on large groups of course can be obtained over 2-3 years.

Löfdahl. You showed this morning that patients with a basal FEV_1 less than -2 SD had the greatest decline by years. How is this decline related to age? This information could be of great importance in planning studies on these patients.

Pride. The rate of annual decline in FEV_1 in both smokers and healthy never-smokers slightly accelerates with increasing age; probably the differences between older smokers and never-smokers increase, but not all studies show this. But in older subjects there are more problems due to cardiovascular disease etc., so there is a trade-off between a bigger signal and more interfering factors.

Arborelius. Several studies have shown that subjects with low FEV_1 % of predicted <u>do</u> die prematurely and mainly not in pulmonary disease, but in the cardiovascular diseases. Hence, it is probably more ethical to try to make smokers stop smoking than to put them on drugs that <u>may</u> counteract deterioration of lung function.

Pride. Of course no drug will be as good as quitting smoking - there are many other risks associated with smoking outside COAD.

Hogg. Would Dr. Bleecker clarify the values of the intervention planned in the American study?

Bleecker. The planning for the American Intervention Study took place 3-5 years ago and at that time pharmacologic interventions centered around the use of bronchodilators. Because of the efficacy of anticholinergic compounds in patients with chronic bronchitis and airflow obstruction, ipratropium was chosen for the pharmacological intervention in the U.S. study. The U.S. study will also examine the effects of smoking on decline in FEV_1. This intervention will remain a major inflammatory and irritant stimulus in these subjects with early airflow obstruction.

Pride. Do you think other tests of responsiveness, which are present in asthmatic but not bronchitic subjects, would be useful in intervention studies? If so, which one?

Hargreave. Yes, challenge tests with stimuli acting indirectly may be useful in subject selection. I don't know which of these stimuli is the best; they include hyperventilation, propranolol, adenosine monophosphate etc.

REFERENCES

Albert, R.K., Martin, T.R., and Lewis, S.W. (1980) Ann. Intern. Med. 92, 753-758.
Anthonisen, N.R., Manfreda, J., Warren, C.P.W., Hershfield, E.S., Harding, G.K.M., and Nelson, N.A. (1987) Ann. Intern. Med. 106, 196-204.
Boman, G., Bäcker, U., Larsson, S., Melander, B., and Wåhlander, L. (1983) Eur. J. Respir. Dis. 64, 405-415.
British Thoracic Society Research Committee. (1985) Thorax 40, 832-835.
Burrows, B., Knudson, R.J., Cline, M.G., and Lebowitz, M.D. (1977) Am. Rev. Respir. Dis. 115, 195-205.
Dockery, D.W., Speizer, F.E., Ferris, B.G. Jr., and Ware, J.H. (1988) Am. Rev. Respir. Dis. 137, 286-292.
Engel, T., Heinig, J.H., Madson, O., Hansen, M., and Weeke, E.R. (1989) Eur. Resp. J. 2, (in press)
Fletcher, C., and Peto, R. (1977) Br. Med. J. 1, 1645-1648.
Higgins, M.W., Keller, J.B., Becker, M., Howatt, W., Landis, J.R., Rotman, H., Weg, J.G., and Higgins, I. (1982) Am. Rev.

Respir. Dis. <u>125</u>, 144-151.
Koëter, G.H., Postma, D.S., De Monchy, J.G.R., Kauffman, H.F., De Vries, K., and Sluiter, H.J. (1989) In: Bronchitis IV, (H.J. Sluiter, R. Van der Lende, J. Gerritsen, and D.S. Postma, Eds.) Groningen, pp 284-294.
Kraan, J., Koëter, G.H., Van der Mark, Th.W., Boorsma, M., Kukler, J., Sluiter, H.J., and De Vries, K. (1988) Am. Rev. Respir. Dis. <u>137</u>, 44-48.
Multicenter Study Group. (1980) Eur. J. Respir. Dis. <u>61</u>, (suppl. 111), 93-108.
Postma, D.S., Stenhuis, E.J., Van der Weele, L.T., and Sluiter, H.J. (1985) Eur. J. Respir. Dis. <u>67</u>, 56-64.
Pride, N.B. (1987) Eur. J. Respir. Dis. <u>7</u>, (suppl. 153), 13-18.
Pride, N.B., Taylor, R.G., Lim. T.K., Joyce, H., and Watson, A. (1987) Bull. Eur. Physiopathol. Respir. <u>23</u>, 369-375.
Stoller, J.K. (1987) Chest <u>91</u>, 155-156.
Stoller, J.K., Gerbarg, Z.B., and Feinstein, A.R. (1987) J. Gen. Intern. Med. <u>2</u>, 29-35.
U.S. Surgeon General. (1984) In: The Health Consequences of Smoking. (U.S. Department of Health and Human Services), pp 76-83.

6) AIRWAYS HYPERREACTIVITY, BRONCHIAL INFLAMMATION AND OBSTRUCTIVE LUNG DISEASE

E.R. Bleecker

Department of Pulmonary and Critical Care Medicine, University of Maryland, School of Medicine, Baltimore, Maryland, USA

SUMMARY: Understanding the mechanisms responsible for the development of chronic airflow obstruction is very important since this disease is the fifth leading cause of death in the United States and it produces a significant economic and social burden for society. Since reversal of established airflow obstruction is not possible, it would appear that the best prognosis and therapeutic results can be obtained by early diagnosis and prevention of irreversible disease. Understanding the underlying pathophysiologic mechanisms is necessary to detect susceptible individuals and develop effective interventions.

INTRODUCTION

Episodic airflow obstruction (asthma) and chronic airflow obstruction (CAO) are not only common disorders but they have many features in common. In some individuals, asthma is characterized by intermittent and reversible airflow obstruction while other asthmatics appear to have pulmonary syndromes that are more progressive and less distinguishable from chronic obstructive lung disease. Often differentiation between asthma and chronic airflow obstruction is complicated by overlapping clinical characteristics (Sluiter & Van der Lende, 1989).

Established definitions of these diseases are descriptive and may not provide insight into the pathogenesis of either asthmatic or chronic airflow obstruction. One approach to understanding the pathogenesis of obstructive airways disease has been to investigate proposed risk factors that are related to their development and severity of airflow obstruction either episodic or chronic. These factors include bronchial hyperreponsiveness, allergy, and environmental exposures (tobacco smoke and air pollutants) which may well interact with each other in the development of obstructive airways disease.

BRONCHIAL HYPERRESPONSIVENESS

One of the most important and consistent findings in subjects with obstructive airways disease is bronchial hyperresponsiveness. This is defined as an exaggerated broncho-constrictor response to various physical, chemical or pharmacologic stimuli (Boushey et al., 1980; Bleecker, 1985; O'Connor et al., 1989). The close association between bronchial hyperresponsiveness and asthma is well established since virtually all asthmatics have elevated levels of nonspecific bronchial hyperresponsiveness (Boushey et al., 1980; Bleecker, 1985). The degree of nonspecific bronchial hyperreactivity distinguishes individuals with allergic rhinitis from those with allergic asthma (Permutt et al., 1977), and cross sectional studies show that the level of bronchial reactivity appears to reflect alterations in symptoms and the clinical severity of asthma (Hargreave et al., 1980).

There has been recent interest in the relationship between bronchial hyperresponsiveness and the development of chronic airflow obstruction (Barter et al., 1976). For example, in asymptomatic sons of subjects with chronic airflow obstruction who were between the ages of 20 to 30 years old, increased airways reactivity was associated with an accelerated loss of pulmonary function (Barter et al., 1976). Postma and co-workers have reported that the decline in FEV_1 over time is closely related to the level of airways responsiveness in individuals with moderate airflow obstruction (Postma et al., 1986). In the Lung Health Study, a multicenter intervention study in the United States funded by the NHLBI, there was a 65 % to 70 % incidence of airways reactivity in 6000 cigarette smokers with mild airflow obstruction (Anthonisen, 1989). Thus, bronchial hyperresponsiveness appears to be related to the development and progression of airflow limitation in subjects with chronic airflow obstruction. Its presence may be an important marker of bronchial inflammation in subjects at risk for the development of chronic airflow obstruction.

The usual mechanisms that have been proposed to explain airways hyperreactivity have emphasized alterations in autonomic neural control of airway tone, the contribution of baseline airflow obstruction, changes in intrinsic bronchial smooth muscle function as well as alterations in bronchial epithelial integrity and permeability. While each of these potential mechanisms may play a role in the development of airways hyperresponsiveness, there is evidence to suggest that bronchial inflammation may be the common factor responsible for the development of this disorder (Nadel, 1984; Bleecker, 1985; Holgate et al., 1987). It is possible that an initial trigger is the release of inflammatory mediators from bronchial mast cells, macrophages, and even, perhaps, epithelial cells which then cause the migration to and activation of inflammatory cells in the airways. These inflammatory changes could then be associated with alterations in epithelial integrity, abnormalities in autonomic neural control, changes in mucociliary function and increased airway smooth muscle responsiveness.

BRONCHIAL INFLAMMATION - IN VITRO STUDIES

One of the major characteristics of immediate hypersensitivity reactions is the development of inflammation. These reactions are caused by the biologic activities of a group of chemical mediators that can be immunologically released from appropriate target cells and organ systems (Austen et al., 1975; Lewis & Austen, 1981). Exposure to a specific antigen in susceptible individuals causes the production of specific reaginic antibody (IgE) which fixes to basophils, mast cells, and other immunologically active cells. Repeat exposure to that antigen then initiates a sequence of cellular biochemical reactions resulting in the release and/or synthesis of mediators such as histamine, prostaglandins, and leukotrienes as well as eosinophil and neutrophil chemotactic factors. These biochemical mediators can produce numerous physiologic and cellular events including contraction of airways smooth muscle, alterations in vascular smooth muscle tone, increased vascular permeability, aggregation and degranulation of platelet, and attraction of inflammatory cells. Thus, an antigenic stimulus that can produce broncho-constriction acutely can also cause chronic inflammation in the airways through a series of immunologic and biochemical reactions (Kaliner, 1984). In addition, recent _in vitro_ evidence suggests that non-immunologic factors such as hyperosmotic stimuli can also cause the release of similar inflammatory mediators (Gravelyn et al., 1988). In man, mediator release is not only dependent on these complex intracellular biochemical interactions, but in addition, they are modulated directly by the local levels of mediators (histamine and prostaglandins), by endogenous levels of hormones and perhaps by autonomic neural reflex pathways (Bleecker, 1986).

These _in vitro_ observations suggest that chemical mediators released from mast cells, basophils or other biologically active cells can cause all of the characteristic physiologic and inflammatory changes associated with asthma (Lewis & Austen, 1981). If correct, there should be obvious associations between situations where there is immunologic mediator release and bronchial inflammation with airways hyperreactivity and airflow obstruction _in vivo_ systems. Increased airways reactivity has been found after environmental and laboratory exposures to specific antigens in allergic asthmatics (Cockcroft et al., 1977;

Golden et al., 1978; Cartier et al., 1982). Usually, increases in non-specific airways responsiveness have been found in asthmatics who have evidence of delayed phase reaction after allergen challenge. Other studies have shown that corticosteroids decreases airways response to histamine in asthmatics (Kerrebijn et al., 1987) and may reduce the levels of increased non-specific airways responsiveness in individuals with occupational asthma (Mapp et al., 1985) or in ragweed allergic asthmatics after aerosolized antigen challenge. In animal models of immediate hypersensitivity reactions, exposure of the airways to antigen is associated with the release of inflammatory mediators as well as increases in the numbers of neutrophils that are found in pulmonary lavage fluid (Bleecker et al., 1985). Delayed immunologic responses when examined in organ systems such as the skin are closely associated with cellular elements that include neutrophils and eosinophils (Poothullil et al., 1976; Schleimer, 1984). Other stimuli such as exposures to infectious agents or airborne pollutants (ozone, SO_2, NO_2) appear to produce their effects by causing inflammation and damage to the airway epithelium (Empey et al., 1976; Holtzman et al., 1983). Interestingly, airways reactivity appears to play an important role in the development of obstructive airway disease in allergic individuals. For example, atopic individuals who do not demonstrate non-specific airways hyperreactivity do not have evidence of clinical asthma (Permutt et al., 1977). However, superficially the association of allergy with asthma and hyperreactivity does not appear to be universal since many adult asthmatics do not appear to have obvious clinical allergies, and one cannot implicate immunologic factors as a basis for their asthma. But, even in these so-called intrinsic asthmatics there is often peripheral blood and sputum eosinophilia, a response associated with allergy and inflammation. It also appears that bronchial reactivity may influence not only the pathogenesis and severity of asthma but may serve as a risk factor for the development of chronic airflow obstruction. Therefore, determining the mechanisms responsible for airways hyperreactivity, its relationship to immunologic factors and inflammation and the ability of drug therapy to modify bronchial hyperresponsiveness are all important approaches necessary for the complete under-standing of the pathophysiology of asthma and chronic obstructive pulmonary disease.

BRONCHIAL INFLAMMATION - IN VIVO STUDIES

A number of approaches have been employed to study these inter-actions in vivo systems. One approach has been the use of animal models that have immunologic characteristics and develop physiologic reactions that are similar to those observed in man. Systemic and local (pulmonary) immediate hypersensitivity reactions have been studied in dogs in our laboratory as well as by other investigators (Lazarus et al., 1979; Hirshman et al., 1983; Bleecker et al., 1985). These studies have demonstrated the release of inflammatory mediators including histamine, leuko-trienes, and prostaglandins systemically as well as locally into respiratory secretions after specific antigen challenge. These immunologic events are associated with characteristic circulatory and respiratory responses as well as an early cellular inflammatory response in the airways (Bleecker et al., 1985). Additional studies that have employed various immunopharmacologic interventions have shown that pretreatment with sympathomimetic agents prevents physiologic changes by blocking mediator release (Silverman et al., 1986) and indomethacin alters the acute physiologic and cellular response to inhaled antigen (Walden et al., 1985). Recent work has localized the physiologic and immunologic responses even further to more peripheral airways by instilling antigen through the tip of a wedged fiberoptic bronchoscope. These studies have shown that there is a signifi-cant relationship between local mediator release and changes in peripheral airways resistance. One of the most important findings by these investigators is the demonstration of mediator release and associated increases in resistance in animals exposed to non-immunologic local airway challenge with dry air administered at high flows through a wedged bronchoscope (Freed et al., 1985). These animal studies define pathologic mechanisms linking immunologic and non-immunologic mediator release with airways inflammation and bronchoconstriction. They also suggest possible approaches for the study of asthma and reactive airway disease in man. However, to fully understand the mechanisms responsible for airway hyperreactivity in asthma and chronic obstructive pulmonary disease, human clinical investigation is necessary.

While the investigation of immunologic and physiologic interactions in man is difficult, recent studies using an _in vivo_ model of human allergic disease have demonstrated the feasibility of this approach (Naclerio et al., 1983). These studies on the pathogenesis of allergic rhinitis have employed a model of local nasal challenge with ragweed antigen in subjects with allergic rhinitis. Briefly they showed that antigen exposure leads to the local release of inflammatory mediators (histamine, kinins, TAME esterase, leukotrienes and prostaglandin D2) into nasal washings (Naclerio et al., 1983; Creticos et al., 1984). The levels of mediators that were released correlated with symptoms such as sneezing and increased nasal airflow resistance. More recent studies have shown that these reactions have a late phase component that is associated with the release of histamine, kinins and TAME esterase but not prostaglandin D2 suggesting a role for the basophil in these delayed reactions (Naclerio et al, 1985). Interestingly, non-immunologic agents such as dry air also cause the release of inflammatory mediators thereby demonstrating mast cell involvement produced by a non-IgE mediated stimulus (Togias et al., 1985). Many of the approaches and procedures used by these investigators can be directly applied to patients with obstructive lung disease through the use of a fiberoptic bronchoscope and bronchoalveolar lavage.

While there are difficulties in studying these interactions in man, recent developments utilizing bronchoalveolar lavage in animal models and in asthmatics make such approaches possible. Bronchoscopic techniques which have been widely used to study inflammatory lung disease permit the characterization of local events in the airways of individuals with asthma and obstructive lung disease. Inflammatory cells obtained by bronchoalveolar lavage appear to be similar to those present in airway tissue, and recent reports indicate that they can be harvested in a viable and functional state (Davis et al., 1982; Martin et al., 1985). In asthma, lavage has been performed safely without complications (National Institutes of Health Workshop Summary, 1985). Studies show that there are increases in eosinophils in bronchoalveolar lavage fluid approximately seven to forty eight hours after an acute antigen challenge (DeMonchy et al., 1985). Local methods for challenging the airways of asthmatics with specific antigen have been developed that are similar to approaches used in animal studies (Metzger et al., 1985). These investigators have observed the local development of erythema and edema in the airways as well as associated changes in inflamma- tory cells 24 to 72 hours after antigen challenge (Metzger et al., 1987). Studies using these techniques have demonstrated elevations in histamine and constrictor proteinoid mediators in asymptomatic asthmatics under baseline conditions (Casale et al., 1987; Liu et al, 1990). More recently local administration of allergen directly into subsegmental airway, cause immediate increases in histamine and constrictor prostenoid mediators in bronchoalveolar lavage fluids (Liu et al, 1988; Wenzel et al., 1989).

Two other methods that have been developed will enhance the ability to study inflammatory airways disease in human subjects. The first employing bronchial biopsies obtained through a bronchoscope was developed by Annika and Lauri Laitinen and their co-workers (Laitinen et al., 1985). They showed evidence of epithelial damage and inflammation in asthmatics with hyperreactive airways. More recently it has been shown that asymptomatic asthmatics have evidence of eosinophilic infiltration and increased collagen deposition in the airway walls (Beasley et al., 1989; Roche et al., 1989). These morphologic approaches are now being used to study the inflammatory events in patients with chronic bronchitis and early obstructive lung disease (Laitinen - personal communication).

Another new method permits direct study of the physiology of the peripheral airways of asthmatics and cigarette smokers with chronic airflow obstruction. Initial studies in asymptomatic asthmatics who have normal baseline pulmonary function and hyperresponsiveness have shown that the resistance to airflow through peripheral airways is an average of 7 to 10 times greater than the resistance of flow through the small airway of normal subjects (Wagner et al., 1990). These changes in peripheral airways resistance were not altered by local administration of a bronchodilator and the increase in resistance correlated with methacholine airways reactivity. Thus, some of the abnormalities in peripheral airway resistance do not appear to involve alterations in smooth muscle function. One may hypothesize that these changes may be produced by inflammation in the small airways. Other studies have investigated peripheral airway resistance in asymptomatic cigarette smokers (Wagner et al., 1989). These studies have shown that some of the smokers had elevated peripheral airway resistance that is similar to that found in asthma. These changes may represent the development of bronchial inflammation and may predict the future development of symptomatic chronic airflow obstruction.

The use of these approaches (bronchial biopsies, bronchoalveolar lavage to measure mediators and cellular events and direct physiologic assessment of airway mechanics) should further our understanding of the interaction between airways hyperresponsive-ness and bronchial inflammation in man. They will permit us to define the role of mediator release in modulating bronchial inflammation and bronchoconstriction and will also allow us to evaluate the effects of various immunopharmacologic interventions. Such insight will improve our general understanding of the pathogenesis of asthma and chronic airflow obstruction and may result in therapeutic approaches useful in these disorders. Furthermore, this work will serve as a basis for the investigation of the relationship between mediator release, airways inflammation and changes in lung mechanics in response to non-immunologic stimuli, thus facilitating a broader understanding of the basic pathologic processes involved in non-allergic obstructive lung disease.

DISCUSSION

Stockley. I notice that the mediators you have measured are present in both smokers and asthmatic lavages in similar concentrations. What do you think this tells us about their putative role in asthma?

Bleecker. The fact that inflammatory mediators are found in both mild asthma and some cigarette smokers appears to support the role of ongoing inflammation in both of these conditions. These patterns differ and not all smokers show deviations of these markers of inflammation. These findings are consistent with the pathogenesis of smoking induced airway disease, e.g. only 15-25 % of cigarette smokers develop symptomatic lung disease.

Stockley. Were the symptomatic asthmatic patients in a stable state or those who rarely have problems?

Bleecker. These asthmatics only required occasional bronchodilators and none had experienced an exacerbation during the last 2 years.

Stockley. Since they are stable, what happens to these measurements during an exacerbation?

Bleecker. We are presently beginning the study of more symptomatic asthmatics.

Persson. It is possible that subjects with allergy but without asthma will also respond with airways cellular mediator release in response to aero-allergen challenges.

Hogg. The peripheral airways and the collateral channels are two resistances in series. Is the increase in resistance due to changes in collateral channels?

Bleecker. We have not studied the specific site of resistance in the asthmatic subjects.

Koëter. What is the reason that pressure increases due to histamine? Is that only due to bronchial smooth muscle contraction?

Bleecker. When we exposed the peripheral airways to an aerosol of histamine that was administered through a wedged bronchoscope, we produced increases in peripheral airway resistance. This response was reversed by the local administration of isoprenaline. This same dose isoprenaline did not reverse completely the increased peripheral airway resistance found under baseline conditions in asthmatics. This finding indicates that even in mild asthmatics there are mechanical abnormalities in the peripheral airways that may be caused by bronchial inflammation and are not due to smooth muscle spasm alone.

Jansen. I was interested in your finding that in experiments comparing local application of allergen compared with installation of pure saline. Recently, at the ATS-meeting, it was shown that influx of cells, especially PMNs might be a result of the procedure itself. Do you know whether neutrophils are active, or are they unimportant in the pathogenesis of the disease? Is this a first lesson to us that the simple presence of cells do not tell us anything about their functional status?

Bleecker. These are very important questions. At present we do not know whether these cellular events are related to the procedure or to the direct or indirect effects of antigen.

Further studies are required to determine whether these cells are active and important in the pathogenesis of asthma.

REFERENCES

Anthonisen, N.J. (1989) Am. Rev. Respir. Dis. 140, 871-872.
Austen, K.F., and Orange, R.P. (1975) Am. Rev. Respir. Dis. 112, 423-426.
Barter, C.E., and Campbell, A.H. (1976) Am. Rev. Respir. Dis. 113, 305-314.
Beasley, R., Roche, W.R., Roberts, J.A., and Holgate, S.T. (1989) Am. Rev. Respir. Dis. 139, 806-817.
Bleecker, E.R. (1985) J. All. Clin. Immun. (1985) 75, 21-24.
Bleecker, E.R. (1986) Am. J. Med. 81, 93-102.
Bleecker, E.R., Walden, S.M., Wagner, E., Peters, S., Kagey-Sobotka, A., Adkinson, N.F. Jr, and Lichtenstein, L.M. (1985) Chest 87, 164-167.
Boushey, H.A., Holtzman, M.J., Sheller, J.R., and Nadel, J.A. (1980) Am. Rev. Respir. Dis. 121, 389-413.
Britt, E.B., Cohen, B., Menkes, H., Bleecker, E.R., Permutt, S., Rosenthal, R., and Norman, P. (1980) Chest 77, 260-261.
Cartier, A., Thomson, N.C., Frith, P.A., Roberts, R., Tech, M., and Hargreave, F.E. (1982) J. All. Clin. Immun. 70, 170-177.
Casale, T.B., Wood, D., Trapp, S., Richerson, H.B., Metzger, W.J., and Hunninghake, G.W. (1987) J. Clin. Invest. 79, 1197-1203.
Cockcroft, D.W., Ruffin, R.E., Dolovich, J., and Hargreave, F.E. (1977) Clin. All. 7, 503-513.
Creticos, P.S., Peters, S.P., Adkinson, N.F. Jr, Naclerio, R.M., Hages, E.C., Norman, P.S., and Lichtenstein L.M. (1984) N. Engl. J. Med. 310, 1626-1630.
Davis, G.S., Giancola, M.S., Costanza, M.C., and Low, R.B. (1982) Am. Rev. Respir. Dis. 126, 611-616.
DeMonchy, J.G.R., Kauffman, H.F., Venge, P., Koeter, G.H., Jansen, H.M., Sluiter, H.J., and DeVries, K. (1985) Am. Rev. Respir. Dis. 131, 373-376.
Empey, D.W., Laitinen, L.A., Jacobs, L., Gold, W.M., and Nadel, J.A. (1976) Am. Rev. Respir. Dis. 113, 131-139.
Freed, A.N., Bromberg-Barnea, B., and Menkes, H.A. (1986) J. Appl. Physiol. 59, 1986-90.
Golden, J.A., Nadel, J.A., and Boushey, H.A. (1978) Am. Rev. Respir. Dis. 118, 287-294.
Gravelyn, T.R., Pan, P.M., and Eschenbacher, W.L. (1988) Am. Rev. Respir. Dis. 1988; 137, 641-646.
Hargreave, F.E., Juniper, E.F., Ryan, G., Dolovich, M., Cartler, A., Frith, P.A., and Newhouse, M.T. (1980) In: Airway Reactivity: Mechanisms and Clinical Relevance. (F.E. Hargreave, Ed) Astra Pharmaceuticals Canada Ltd., pp. 216-221.
Hirshman, C.A., Peters, J., Butler, J., Hanifin, J.M., and

Downes, H. (1983) J. Appl. Physiol. $\underline{54}$, 1108-1114.
Holgate, S.T., Beasley, R., and Twentyman, O.P. (1987) Clin. Sci. $\underline{73}$, 561-572.
Holtzman, M.J., Fabbri, L.M., O'Byrne, P.M., Gold, B.D., Aizawa, H., Walters, E.H., Alpert, S.E., and Nadel, J.A. (1983) Am. Rev. Respir. Dis. $\underline{127}$, 686-690.
Kaliner, M. (1984) J. All. Clin. Immun. $\underline{73}$, 311-315.
Kerrebijn, K.F., van Essen-Zandvliet, E.E.M., and Neijens, H.J. (1987) J. All. Clin. Immun. $\underline{79}$, 653-659.
Laitinen, L.A., Heino, M., Laitinen, A., Kava, T., and Haahtela, T. (1985) Am. Rev. Respir. Dis. $\underline{31}$, 599-606.
Lazarus, S.C., Chesrown, S.E., Frey, M.J., Reed, B.R., Mjorndal, T.O., and Gold, W.M. (1979) J. Appl. Physiol. $\underline{46}$, 919-926.
Lewis, R.A., and Austen, K.F. (1981) Nature (London) $\underline{293}$, 103-108.
Liu, M.C., Hubbard, W., McLemore, T., Kagey-Sobotka, A., Lichtenstein, L., and Bleecker, E.R. (1988) Clin. Res. $\underline{36}$, 507..
Liu, M.C., Bleecker, E.R., Lichtenstein, L.M., Kagey-Sobotka, A., Niv, Y., McLemore, T.L., Permutt, S., Proud, D., and Hubbard, W.C. (1990) Am. Rev. Respir. Dis. $\underline{141}$, in press.
Mapp, C.E., Polato, R., Maestrelli, P., Hendrick, D.J., and Fabbri, L.M. (1985) J. All. Clin. Immun. $\underline{75}$, 568-572.
Martin, T.R., Raghu, G., Maunder, R.J., and Springmeyer, S.C. (1985) Am. Rev. Respir. Dis. $\underline{132}$, 254-260.
Metzger, W.J., Nugent, K., Richerson, H.B., Moseley, P., Lakin, R., Zavala, D., and Hunninghake, G.W. (1985) Chest $\underline{87}$, 165-195.
Metzger, W.J., Zavala, D., Richerson, H.B., Moseley, P., Iwamota, P., Monick, M., Sjoerdsma, K.W., and Hunninghake, G.W. (1987) Am. Rev. Respir. Dis. $\underline{135}$, 433-440.
Naclerio, R.M., Meier, H.L., Kagey-Sobotka, A., Adkinson, N.F. Jr, Meyers, D.A., Norman, P.S., and Lichtenstein, L.M. (1983) Am. Rev. Respir. Dis. $\underline{128}$, 597-601.
Naclerio, R.M., Proud, D., Togias, A.G., Adkinson, N.F. Jr, Meyers, D.A., Kagey-Sobotka, A., Plaut, M., Norman, P.S., and Lichtenstein, L.M. (1985) N. Engl. J. Med. $\underline{313}$, 65-70.
Nadel, J.A. (1984) J. All. Clin. Immun. $\underline{73}$, 651-652.
National Institutes of Health Workshop Summary. (1985) J. All. Clin. Immun. $\underline{76}$, 145-147.
O'Connor, G.T., Sparrow, D., and Weiss, S.T. (1989) Am. Rev. Respir. Dis. $\underline{140}$, 225-252.
Permutt, S., Rosenthal, R.R., Norman, P.S., and Menkes, H.A. (1977) In: Asthma, Physiology, Immunopharmacology and Treatment. (L.M. Lichtenstein and K.F. Austin, Eds) Academic Press, New York, pp. 265-282.
Poothullil, J., Umemoto, L., Dolovich, J., Hargreave, F.E., and Day, R.P. (1976) J. All. Clin. Immun. $\underline{57}$, 164-167.
Postma, D.S., De Vries, K., Koëter, G.H., and Sluiter, H.J. (1986) Am. Rev. Respir. Dis. $\underline{134}$, 276-280.
Roche, R., Beasley, R., Williams, J.H., and Holgate, S.T. (1989) Lancet $\underline{1}$, 520-524.
Schleimer, R.P. (1984) Ann. Rev. Pharm. $\underline{25}$, 384-411.
Silverman, H.J., Taylor, W.R., Smith, P.L., Kagey-Sobotka, A., Lichtenstein, L.M., and Bleecker, E.R. (1986) Am. Rev. Respir.

Dis. <u>134</u>, 243-247.
Sluiter, H.J., VanDerLende, R. (1989) In: Bronchitis IV. Royal
    Vangorcum Assn Ltd. The Netherlands.
Togias, A.G., Naclerio, R.M., Proud, D., Fish, J.E., Adkinson,
    N.F. Jr., Kagey-Sobotka, A., Norman, P.S., and Lichtenstein
    LM. (1985) J. Clin. Invest. <u>76</u>, 1375-1381.
Wagner, E.M., Liu, M.C., Permutt, S., and Bleecker, E.R. (1989)
    Am. Rev. Respir. Dis. <u>139</u>, (4/2), A108.
Wagner, E.M., Liu, M.C., Weinmann, G.G., Permutt, S., and
    Bleecker, E.R. (1990) Am. Rev. Respir. Dis. <u>141</u>, 584-588.
Walden, S.M., Peters, S., Adkinson, N.F., and Bleecker, E.R.
    (1985) Am. Rev. Respir. Dis. <u>131</u>, (4/2), A29-.
Wenzel, S.E., Westcott, J.Y., Smith, H.R., and Larsen, G.L.
    (1989) Am. Rev. Respir. Dis. <u>139</u>, 450-457.

7) CLINICAL TRIALS IN ASTHMA AND CHRONIC AIRFLOW OBSTRUCTION

Deborah A. Meyers[1], and E.R. Bleecker[2]

[1]Departments of Medicine and Epidemiology, The Johns Hopkins University, School of Medicine and School of Hygiene and Public Health; [2]Department of Medicine, Division of Pulmonary and Critical Care Medicine, University of Maryland, School of Medicine, Baltimore, Maryland, USA

SUMMARY: Clinical trials are becoming increasingly important in objectively evaluating therapeutic interventions in pulmonary medicine. Although the overall methodology for clinical trials is similar for most diseases, there are specific questions and problems unique to pulmonary medicine. This review is limited to a discussion of the general design and commonly encountered "problems and pitfalls" for clinical trials in respiratory medicine. Three examples of designs for intervention in asthma and chronic obstructive airways disease are presented.

INTRODUCTION

Clinical trials in asthma and chronic airflow obstruction provide important mechanisms to evaluate different therapeutic modalities (Pocock, 1983; Meinert, 1986). They range from studies on the effectiveness of a bronchodilator or anti-inflammatory agent to non-pharmacologic interventions such as the evaluation of oxygen therapy (Anthonisen, 1983; Kerrebijn et al., 1987; Barnes, 1989). Other studies may investigate the effects of changes in lifestyle that may include smoking cessation or the avoidance of exposure to environmental or occupational provoking agents (Anthonisen, 1989).

Clinical trials provide a valid scientific approach to investigate not only new forms of therapy but they provide essential data used by governmental regulatory agencies and the pharmaceutical industry for new drug development. Thus, well designed clinical trials have a wider role in clinical medicine. They can be used not only to assess the efficacy of new approaches but also to reevaluate current or accepted forms of therapy objectively, proving or disproving the value of that treatment modality (Mckhann, 1989). Furthermore, results from clinical trials often provide important insights into the pathophysiology of a disease process and may lead to new indications for a specific therapeutic regimen.

Ideally, clinical trials should employ objective endpoints to assess the effects of a specific intervention. When objective parameters cannot be measured, it is necessary to rely on more subjective parameters such as changes in respiratory symptoms or decreases in co-medication use as primary endpoints. However, assessment of symptom severity can be improved by employing validated symptom-medication diaries and constantly attempting to determine how these subjective endpoints correlate with more objective parameters. Furthermore, the use of study medications and co-medications, can be quantified by utilizing computerized pill counters or a microprocessor system that records the time and number of each nebulizer activation (Spector et al., 1986; Rand, 1989).

The purpose of this paper will be to provide an outline and summary of the specific features that need to be considered in the development, organization, and completion of clinical trials in subjects with obstructive lung disease. These principles are outlined in Table I. Examples of clinical trials in asthma and chronic airflow obstruction will be used throughout this review to illustrate some of the issues that arise in their design and execution.

Table I. Protocol Design and Development

I   Study Objectives and Specific Aims

II   Recruitment
          Medical Sources
          Media Advertisement
          Mass Screening

III   Characterization
          Clinical Evaluation
          Pulmonary Function
          Airways Responsiveness
          Experimental Techniques (Bronchoscopy)

IV   Interventions
          Behavioral (Smoking Cessation)
          Pharmacologic
            Bronchodilator
            Anti-inflammatory
          Other
            Environmental Modification

V   Compliance
          Subject Selection
          Investigator Involvement
          Objective Monitoring
          Behavioral Techniques
          Reward System

VI   Quality Assurance
          Double Blind Experimental Conditions
          Detailed Standardized Procedures
          Periodic Site Visits
          Independent Quality Control

VII   Assessment
          Objective Endpoints
             Pulmonary Function (spirometry)
             Peak Expiratory Flow Rates
             Airways Reactivity

          Subjective Endpoints
             Clinical Status
             Symptoms/Co-medication use
             Quality of Life

          New Experimental Approaches
             Bronchoscopic Procedures

VIII   Data Management and Analysis
          Centralized Data Center
          Communications Network (FAX)

contd /...

        Well Designed Data Collection Forms
        Computerized Data Entry
        Efficient and Timely Analysis
        Independent Interim Analysis and Safety Monitoring

The first example will be a study to determine whether a therapeutic agent can acutely effect airways reactivity. Non-specific bronchial reactivity is thought to reflect underlying bronchial inflammation in asthma (Bleecker, 1984; Nadel, 1984; Holgate, 1987). Thus, evaluating the effects of a therapeutic agent on non-specific or allergen induced bronchial responses provides an objective means to profile the spectrum of activity of both bronchodilators as well as non-bronchodilator, anti-asthma compounds. The specific example that will be used in this review is whether an agent can reduce or block exercise induced asthma. This type of study is clearly one of the easiest to design, perform, and complete. While there are clear, easily defined endpoints in these studies, there may not be a direct relationship between pharmacologic effects on airway reactivity and an agent's subsequent clinical efficacy. However, these acute laboratory studies are often viewed as an initial step in the development of a new therapeutic agent in man.

The second is a study to determine whether a non-bronchodilator anti-asthma agent has clinical efficacy and improves asthmatic symptoms and/or pulmonary function over time. These trials are more complicated to perform, usually demand a multicenter design, require a number of months of clinical follow-up and often rely on more subjective endpoints. Because of the larger sample size required, they are more costly to perform and they require a more substantial commitment from both the investigators and study participants.

The third trial represents a more recent development in the approach to the treatment of chronic airflow obstruction. The trial may be employed to study interventions that are performed early in the course of chronic obstructive pulmonary disease. The purpose of this clinical trial, is to determine whether a therapeutic intervention improves pulmonary function and alters the natural history and progression of chronic airflow obstruction (Fletcher & Peto, 1977). Since airways hyper-responsiveness and presumably bronchial inflammation are found in subjects with early chronic airflow obstruction, a primary endpoint may also be the reduction of airways hyperreactivity (Barter & Campbell, 1976; Britt et al., 1980; Postma et al., 1986; O'Connor et al., 1989). These trials are more difficult to perform because the primary endpoint is a reduction in the decline in pulmonary function (FEV_1) over time. Long term follow-up is necessary because chronic airflow obstruction may follow a variable course. Decline in pulmonary function may occur gradually over the entire course of this disease or it is possible that larger declines in FEV_1 may be interspersed with more stable periods of airway function. Because of these issues, sample size increases and large numbers of subjects need to be screened. However, these attempts at early intervention in chronic airflow obstruction are important because it may be possible to prevent the development of this common disease process that is associated with significant morbidity and mortality (Anthonisen, 1989).

STUDY OBJECTIVES

First, the purpose of the study must be clearly stated in both a general and specific format. The relevance and importance of the study objectives as well as the ability to accurately answer these questions need to be addressed. Ideally, study objectives should be based on hypotheses that are related to pathophysio-logic mechanisms of the specific disease under investigation.

For the first trial, the general purpose is to determine whether a drug blocks exercise-induced asthma better than a placebo in subjects with asthma (Fig. 1). In the second trial, the general purpose is to determine whether a new drug improves asthmatic symptoms as well as associated objective parameters e.g. diurnal peak expiratory flow rates and/or airways reactivity

(Fig. 2). In the third trial, it is to determine whether a drug improves or reduces the decline in pulmonary function and/or airways hyper-reactivity in patients with chronic airflow obstruction (Fig. 3).

Next the question must be answered; what are the specific primary outcome variables? These endpoints need to be defined during the initial phases of study design prior to testing and randomization of subjects. Clear presentation of primary and secondary endpoints is necessary to design and perform subsequent data analysis. Also these endpoints will be used during interim analysis in long term trials to determine whether positive and/or adverse therapeutic effects dictate early study cessation because

Purpose: To determine whether a drug blocks exercise-induced
                bronchospasm in asthmatic patients

Endpoint: Peak fall in FEV_1 during exercise challenge compared
                to the corresponding peak fall when the patient is on
                placebo

Crossover   Patients with known bronchospasm after exercise challenge,
Design: double-blind, one center

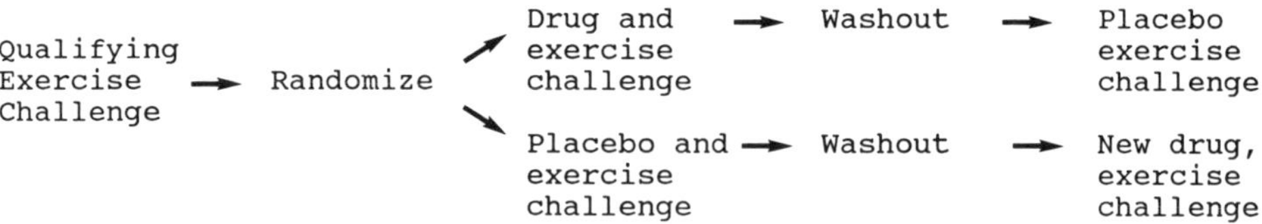

Figure 1. Trial 1

of medical or ethical issues. Thus, development of primary and secondary endpoints are necessary in order to precisely focus the purpose of the study, determine appropriate methods of data analysis and allow calculation of sample size.

As illustrated in Figure 1, for the first trial which is a pulmonary laboratory based trial on the effects of a new drug on exercise-induced asthma, objective endpoints can be easily defined. These outcome variables can be clearly stated e.g. reduction in the peak fall of FEV_1 or in the duration of reduced pulmonary function (area under curve) after exercise compared to the corresponding change in pulmonary function when the subject is pretreated with a placebo.

Purpose: To determine whether a non-bronchodilator anti-asthmatic
                agent improves asthmatic symptoms (and peak flow rates)
                compared to placebo

Endpoint: Decrease in symptom-medication scores

Parallel   2 groups of asthmatic patients (matched for age, sex),
Design: double-blind, multicenter

Screening → Baseline → Randomization → Record symptoms and
                       (drug or   medication use,
                       placebo)   measure peak flow
                                        rates

Figure 2.   Trial 2

For the second trial, there are both objective and subjective measurements, either of which in specific cases may comprise the primary outcome. While measurement of objective endpoints is preferable, drugs employed in these trials may not be bronchodilators and changes in pulmonary function may not occur especially when asthmatics with normal or near normal pulmonary function are studied. While theoretically these agents should improve non-specific airways reactivity and daily variation in peak expiratory flow rates, symptomatic improvement as measured by symptom diaries and the use of co-medications may be the major measures of efficacy.

Purpose: To determine whether a drug slows the decline in
            pulmonary function and improves airways reactivity
            in patients with early chronic obstructive lung disease

Endpoint: Changes in pulmonary function (and airways reactivity)
            over a period of several years

Parallel
Design: 2 groups of patients, double-blind, multicenter study

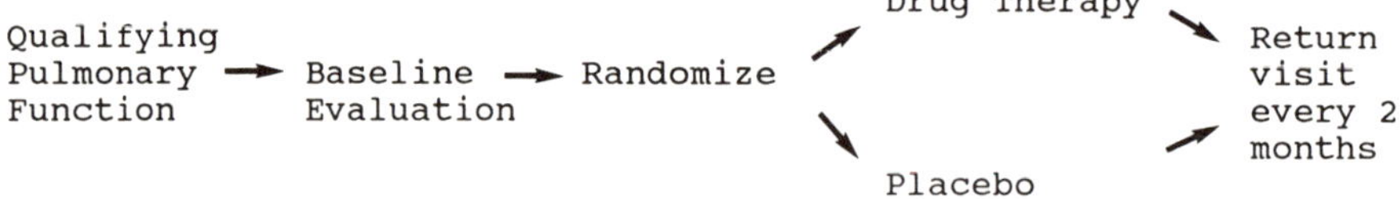

Figure 3.   Trial 3

For the third trial, the primary outcome variables are objective: either an improvement in pulmonary function before and/or after treatment, a decrease in non-specific airways reactivity, or a more difficult endpoint to assess: the reduction in the decline in lung function over a period of time lasting several years. In addition to these objective parameters, factors related to quality of life may be evaluated. However, improvement in subjective function may be difficult to document especially if subjects with early airflow obstruction are studied.

STUDY DESIGN

Design of the clinical trial is often time-consuming and should be viewed as a team approach. It requires cooperation between sponsoring agencies (government or industry), statistical, epidemiologic and clinical investigators. Study design needs to be completed prior to subject enrollment. Subsequent amendments need to be documented with the date and rationale for any changes in protocol. These changes require approval by all principal investigators. Usually a double blind trial is preferable to a single blind design. Occasionally, information contained either in the consent form or the nature of intervention itself (e.g. surgery or smoking cessation) may effect the ability to maintain a strict double blind study design. Choosing between a crossover or parallel design would be determined based on the type and duration of the study under development.

The first study would be a crossover double blind trial. One group of subjects with a previously characterized exercise response would be randomized to receive either the drug or the placebo first. After a sufficient washout period, the subjects would be treated with the other medication and another exercise challenge performed. An issue that often arises is the duration of therapy prior to exercise or other bronchial challenge: should treatment consist of a single drug dose or therapy that is maintained for one or more days prior to bronchial challenge?

This question is important in the evaluation of nonbronchodilator anti-asthma drugs that may not acutely effect airways reactivity but may require more prolonged therapy to produce an effect. With longer pre-challenge dosing schedules, a sufficient washout period must be employed to abolish potential residual drug effects. With other challenges, specifically allergen, the interval between studies must be long enough so that potential delayed effects of allergen exposure on non-specific airways reactivity do not effect the results of subsequent bronchial challenge.

The second and third studies would both have a parallel design; that is, two groups of subjects would be studied where one group receives the study medication and the other receives a placebo drug. This would be performed in a double-blind manner; neither the subjects nor the investigators would know which intervention an individual is receiving. Subjects would be randomized to a specific treatment group. One dose of drug would be studied. Although it is possible to have groups of patients receiving different drug dosages to establish a dose response relationship, this is difficult to preform because of the very large sample size required. If necessary randomization could be stratified for age, and perhaps other specific clinical factors such as allergic status, smoking or medication use. Stratification that is based on too many factors is not feasible or necessary, if patients are assigned to a specific intervention in a random manner.

These last two studies would usually be designed as multicenter trials, while the first study could be performed in a single laboratory with other laboratories performing similar studies using different challenge procedures. There are several obvious advantages to multicenter trials; a larger number of subjects often with diverse clinical, environmental or social backgrounds can be screened, recruited and studied in a shorter period of time. Thus, the conclusions may be applicable to a broader range of patients. There are also disadvantages; the administration of the study and data collection procedures are more complicated. All investigators must strictly follow the same protocol. Specific methods must be rigorously standardized and these procedures followed even if there are individual disagreements with specific aspects of the protocol. Multicenter studies require more initial preparation time; monitoring of each center to assure uniform procedures; and data analysis may require an independent statistical center. In addition in some studies, other geographic factors such as seasonal and environmental exposures to allergens or air pollutants could be important and should be taken into account to prevent additional confounding factors that may be difficult to incorporate into the data analysis.

STUDY POPULATION

Obviously, the first general question that must be addressed is the recruitment and screening of appropriate subjects. Subjects can be recruited through specific medical contacts, media advertisement or general mass screening. Depending on the number and specific characteristics of subjects required, different recruitment strategies will be needed.

The first trial will be based in a single laboratory, the investigators conducting the study may have a sufficient registry of well characterized subjects to complete enrollment. The second trial will be a larger trial and involve multiple centers. Media advertisements as well as regional contacts with local physicians could be used to recruit patients. However, the third large multicenter study of early intervention in chronic airflow obstruction may require screening of a large number of subjects who have such mild symptoms that they may be unaware of the diagnosis of early airflow obstruction. Widespread media advertisement will be necessary; however, non-specific mailings using general mailing lists may not be cost effective. It is possible to obtain complete lists of voters in a specific geographic area, employees of a local large company or individuals who have a certain types of health insurance. In some of these population groups specific characteristics (age, sex, geographic location) as well as risk factors (cigarette smoking, occupation) may be determined prior to screening. The cost benefit of such an approach must be carefully considered. More general approaches are useful, if the study is large and its aim is to learn about the prevalence and natural history of this disease process as well as to intervene in subjects with very early evidence of airflow obstruction.

Before potential subjects can be screened, definition of the specific disease and its severity must be clearly stated. If possible, standardized definitions developed in consensus statements such as, those from the American Thoracic Society's or the Societas Europea Pneumologica should be employed (Snider et al., 1985). However, it will be necessary to delineate specific clinical characteristics of study subjects in terms of their medical history, smoking status, prior use of medication, pulmonary function and overall clinical status. Specific exclusion criteria e.g. medical conditions which would prevent a patient from enrolling in a study based on safety, potential interactions with concomitant medications or other confounding variables need to be clearly stated. Routine and experimental laboratory evaluations that may be employed to test subjects are listed in Table II (Chatham et al., 1982; Laitinen et al., 1985; American Thoracic Society, 1987; Beasley et al., 1989; Liu et al., 1990; Wagner et al., 1990). The results from such testing will be used to characterize subjects as well as to serve as endpoints to assess efficacy of the intervention. The completeness and complexity of laboratory assessment will be determined by available expertise, subject and investigator time constraints, the experimental nature of the specific testing procedures employed, and economic issues that arise when large numbers of subjects require evaluation.

Table II.   Airways Responsiveness and Specialized Pulmonary Evaluation

Bronchial Challenges:

1. Non-specific Airways Reactivity

    A. Methacholine, histamine
    B. Exercise, isocapneic hyperventilation
    C. Osmotic challenges (hypo- or hypertonic solutions)
    D. SO_2

2. Specific agents

    A. Allergen
    B. Prostaglandins (PGD_2)
    C. Leukotrienes
    D. Adenosine, AMP
    E. Bradykinin, Neuropeptides

Bronchoscopic techniques:

1. Bronchial biopsy (morphologic studies)

2. Bronchoalveolar Lavage Techniques:

    A. Cell numbers and differential
    B. Mediator levels
    C. "In vitro" cell function

Physiology:

1. Airways mechanics
   Standard pulmonary function testing

2. Specialized techniques
   Direct and indirect measurements of peripheral airways function

INTERVENTIONS

The specific interventions and experimental protocol must be defined before the experimental studies are undertaken. The overall goal will be to objectively evaluate an intervention that will improve respiratory symptoms, pulmonary function or alter the natural history of the disease under investigation. The specifics of the intervention will depend on the overall objectives of the trial and various approaches are discussed in the examples described below.

For the first study, a straightforward crossover design will be used. The washout interval will be determined by the duration of action of the therapy, and whether the challenge produced delayed or prolonged effects (allergen) between study days. In a double blind random manner, the patient will ingest the drug or placebo under supervision prior to the exercise challenge. All challenges will be performed using the same protocol at the same time of day, subjects must not have taken other specific drugs (bronchodilators, theophylline, caffeine containing beverages, or anti-inflammatory agents) within a given period of time before the exercise studies. This type of study can be performed relatively quickly, and may represent an important early step in the decision whether to continue development of a new drug.

The second study will take approximately two to four months to complete. After qualifying, all subjects will enter a baseline period where they will use only the approved co-medications and fill out a daily symptom-medication diary. Patients will also record their morning and evening peak expiratory flow rates and list all concurrent medication use. Examples of the types of questions that would comprise a symptom-medication diary are illustrated in Table III. The data from the last two weeks of this period will serve as baseline data. Following this period, the patients will be randomized to either the placebo or an active drug group and will follow the same procedures for a predetermined number of weeks. In some trials, the study may be continued for as long as one year. Alternatives to this approach would be to determine whether the new agent can be substituted for an existing drug regimen. In this situation the drug that is being replaced can be withdrawn during the course of the trial, and symptoms and pulmonary function followed. When necessary, the study physician may prescribe additional drugs in a predetermined manner to control asthmatic symptoms. A device that monitors study medications as well as co-medication use could be used to objectively assess compliance.

The third study is one in which the value of early treatment of a chronic and progressive disease is evaluated. Interventions may consist of bronchodilator therapy, early treatment with anti-inflammatory compounds such as inhaled corticosteroids. These may be evaluated alone or may be combined with non-pharmacologic therapies such as smoking cessation.

Table III. Components of Symptom/Co-medication Diary

Assessment of Daytime Asthma Severity:

    A. Symptoms

        1. Shortness of Breath/Chest Tightness
        2. Wheeze
        3. Cough

    B. Overall evaluation of daytime Asthma symptoms

Assessment of Nighttime Asthma Severity

    A. Symptoms

        1. Shortness of breath/Chest Tightness
        2. Wheeze
        3. Cough

    B. Overall evaluation of whether asthma disturbed sleep pattern

Number, Frequency and Severity of Asthma Attacks

Morning and Evening Peak Expiratory Flow Rate Determinations

Record of Use of Study and/Other Medications

Quality of Life:

    Absences due to asthma from work, school, or vacation

    Presence of associated medical conditions: upper respiratory tract infections, sinusitis, rhinitis

CRITERIA FOR EVALUATION OF STUDY RESULTS

Compliance on the part of the investigators and subjects is essential. Study center personnel must adhere to the experimental procedures and maintain the double blind experimental design.

Obviously, subjects who have difficulties keeping appointments during the screening or baseline period should not be enrolled in the study. Investigator involvement is often a crucial factor, and the nurse clinician or technician preforming the studies must be readily accessible to the subjects. Objective monitoring of compliance with the study protocol whenever possible is very useful. Small microprocessors that record the time and usage of the study medication are commercially available (Spector et al., 1986). Weighing of the nebulizer and pill counting are useful but provide less objective methods to assess compliance. For example, recent monitoring of subjects enrolled in a large multi-center therapeutic trial in chronic obstructive lung disease demonstrated that a number of subjects willfully emptied their metered dose inhalers prior to follow-up (Rand et al., 1989). Canister weighing in these individuals would show excellent compliance, while in reality these subjects were not using their medications reliably. If diary forms are used, they should be returned and reviewed for accuracy every two to four weeks rather than at the end of the trial. Volunteer fees should be considered and in long term studies, different reward systems (social gatherings, raffles, certificates for attendance and study completion etc.) are very useful in maintaining compliance at a high level.

QUALITY ASSURANCE

Quality assurance procedures need to be defined in the protocol and implemented before the actual study begins. In multicenter studies, testing procedures should be monitored in each center to insure that all centers are performing evaluations in the same manner, that data is being rigorously collected and appropriate blinding is maintained. Periodic site visits from a central coordinating group or an independent agency provide a very useful mechanism to monitor each study site. Obvious items that should be reviewed would include, the availability of equipment and its calibration, ability of personnel to perform accurate testing and actual review of the raw experimental results. Any deviation from the protocol must be carefully documented. The date and reasons for any amendments must become part of the experimental protocol. Data entry and verification procedures should be standardized and computer software programs should be designed to check for consistency of experimental data.

DATA MANAGEMENT AND ANALYSIS

Data management and analysis needs to be carefully planned before any study is begun. The involvement of investigators with expertise in study design and statistics during the initial stages of study development is necessary. There is often a data management center for large multicenter studies where all data is received and independently analyzed. In such situations, it is important that appropriate computer and fax communication networks exist to provide rapid and accurate data transfer.

Data collection forms must be clear, concise, and easy to follow. Each form should include instructions to assure that they can be accurately completed. This is especially important for symptom-medication diaries which are filled out by study participants. Although symptom-medication diaries are commonly used, it is still desirable to validate a specific symptom-medication diary.

As previously discussed, primary endpoints and the methods of analysis must be determined prior to starting the study. For long-term studies, interim analysis may be performed at a predetermined stage of the study. A group of independent reviewers should be used; since it will be necessary for them to discuss the current results without regard to the double blinding procedure. If the trial is discontinued early because of the results of the interim analysis, the 'stopping rules' need to be clearly stated in the protocol before the start of the trial. Of course, it is also important to plan the statistical analysis in such a manner so that results of the trial will be available in a timely fashion after the conclusion of the study.

It is not within the scope of this paper to present detailed statistical methodology but several points should be stressed. Statistical involvement is not only required for data analysis when the study is completed but is necessary throughout the period of study design. However, medical expertise must be used to determine the magnitude of the treatment effects that would be clinically significant. Clinical investigators must also familiarize the statisticians with the type of data that will be collected including sources of potential errors. That will allow decisions to be made as to the type of analyses that should be performed (for example, parametric: t-test, ANOVA or non-parametric: rank tests, chi-squared test). During the planning stages, it is necessary to calculate the sample size needed to ensure that meaningful study results can be expected when the study is completed. This calculation is based on the expected results: magnitude of the difference between the treatment and the amount of variance. The expected difference between treatment groups is often based on what is considered clinically significant while the variance is estimated from previous studies in the same area.

The first trial is the most straightforward of the three trials. A clinically significant result might be a peak fall in FEV_1 during exercise challenge of at least 10 percentage points less than the corresponding peak fall when the patient receives a placebo. Since early bronchoprovocation studies can be pivotal in the decision process during drug development, it may be desirable to calculate sample size based on a statistical power of 90 % with a significance level of 0.01. In this case, a decision may be made not to continue further development and testing if the drug does not produce obvious effects on airways reactivity.

For the second trial, if differences in symptom-medication scores are the primary endpoints, a decrease of 30 % in scores between the treated and placebo group may be considered clinically significant. Sample size calculations could be based on commonly used values, a power of 80 % with a significance level of 0.05. This is usually based on a 2-tailed test, although one could argue that a 1-tailed test is appropriate, since there may be no reason to believe that the drug would worsen asthma symptoms. If a 1-tail test is used, a smaller sample size could be used. Although a 1-tail test may be justified based on statistical reasoning, regulatory agencies and scientific journals may require using a 2-tailed test.

The third trial may well involve hundreds of patients studied in a number of different centers. Any study of intervention in the early stages of a progressive disease would usually involve a larger number of patients than intervention studies performed in more symptomatic patients. The goal is to demonstrate that the proposed intervention produces a significant result; however, these patients only have evidence of "mild" disease, may be characterized by more random variation in symptoms and respiratory function, and the difference that is expected between study groups may be small in magnitude. Therefore, it will be necessary to study a large group of patients to demonstrate statistical significance.

It is also necessary to decide on secondary endpoints and their method of analysis before the trial is begun. This should be documented in the experimental protocol. There may well be multiple secondary endpoints; some of them may be often exploratory in nature. However, significant results in these secondary analyses may be useful in planning future studies. If changes in a secondary endpoint are documented in one trial, these measurements may be chosen as a primary endpoints in subsequent studies. Other parameters that are investigated may be useful in understanding the basic disease processes. For example, improvement in airways reactivity may result from increases in baseline pulmonary function or decreases in bronchial inflammation. It is important that appropriate statistical analysis of secondary endpoints is employed, since multiple tests are being performed that may lead to the false impression of significant results. Of course, it is important to remember that significance levels of 0.05 or 0.01 are not absolute; other levels (higher or lower) may be chosen for appropriate reasons. In some cases, a significance level between 0.05 and 0.10 may be considered adequate to continue further testing of a new drug.

CONCLUSION: The general design of clinical trials for the evaluation of obstructive airways disease have been presented. The types of trials range from simple laboratory based procedures to complex clinical studies that may take several years to complete. The importance of extensive planning and discussion with both clinical and statistical investigators as well as individuals from regulatory agencies has been stressed. This approach is necessary in order to develop a well defined study design that will allow the investigator to obtain accurate experimental data.

Acknowledgment: We wish to thank Elizabeth Walters for her secretarial assistance in the preparation of this manuscript.

REFERENCES

American Thoracic Society. (1987) Am. Rev. Respir. Dis. <u>136</u>, 1285-1298.
Anthonisen, N.R. (1983) Ann. Intern. Med. <u>99</u>, 519-527.
Anthonisen, N.J. (1989) Am. Rev. Respir. Dis. <u>140</u>, 871-872.
Barnes, P.J. (1989) N. Eng. J. Med. <u>321</u>, 1517-1527.
Barter, C.E., and Campbell, A.H. (1976) Am. Rev. Resp. Dis. <u>113</u>, 305-314.
Beasley, R., Roche, W.R., Roberts, J.A., and Holgate, S.T. (1989) Am. Rev. Respir. Dis. <u>139</u>, 806-817.
Bleecker, E.R. (1984) J. Allergy & Clin. Immun. <u>75</u>, 21-24.
Britt, E.B., Cohen, B., Menkes, H., Bleecker, E.R., Permutt, S., Rosenthal, R., and Norman, P. (1980) Chest <u>77</u>, 260-261.
Chatham, M., Bleecker, E.R., Smith, P.L., Rosenthal, R.R., Mason P., and Norman, P.S. (1982) Am. Rev. Respir. Dis. <u>126</u>, 235-240.
Fletcher, C., and Peto, R. (1977) Br. Med. J. <u>1</u>, 1645-1648.
Holgate, S.T., Beasley, R., and Twentyman, O.P. (1987) Clin. Sci. <u>73</u>, 561-572.
Kerrebijn, K.F., van Essen-Zandvliet, E.E.M., and Neijens, H.J. (1987) J. All. Clin. Immunol. <u>79</u>, 653-659.

Laitinen, L.A., Heino, M., Laitinen, A., Kava, T., and Haahtela,
    T. (1985) Am. Rev. Respir. Dis. 131, 599-606.
Liu, M.C., Bleecker, E.R., Niv, Y., Kagey-Sobotka, A., McLemore,
    T.L., Permutt, S., Lichtenstein, L.M., Proud, D., and Hubbard,
    W.C. (1990) Am. Rev. Resp. Dis. 142 (in press).
Mckhann, GM. (1989) Archives of Neurology 46, 611-614.
Meinert, CL. (1986) Oxford Univ Press, New York.
Nadel, J.A. (1984) J. All. Clin. Immunol. 73, 651-653.
O'Connor, G.T., Sparrow, D., and Weiss, S.T. (1989) Am. Rev.
    Respir. Dis. 140, 225-252.
Pocock, S.J. (1983) In: Clinical Trials. John Wiley and Sons, New
    York.
Postma, D.S., De Vries, K., Koeter, G.H., and Sluiter, H.J.
    (1986) Am. Rev. Respir. Dis. 134, 276-280.
Rand, C.S., Tashkin, D., Wise, R.A., Nides, M., Simon, M., and
Bleecker, E.R. (1989) Am. Rev. Respir. Dis. 139, (4/2): A16
Spector, S.L., Kinsman, R., Mawhinney, H., Siegel, S.C.,
    Rachelefsky, G.S., Katz, R.M., and Rohr, A.L. (1986) J. All.
    Clin. Imm. 77, 65-70.
Snider, G.L., Kleinerman, J., Thurlbeck, W.M., and Bengali, Z.H.
    (1985) Am. Rev. Respir. Dis. 132, 182-185.
Wagner, E.M., Weinmann, G.G., Liu, M.C., and Bleecker, E.R.
    (1990) Am. Rev. Respir. Dis. 142, (in press).

8)   A CRITICAL LOOK AT BLOOD SAMPLES IN CB AND COAD

P. Venge

Laboratory for Inflammation Research, Department of Clinical
Chemistry, University Hospital, S-751 85 Uppsala, Sweden

SUMMARY: Few studies have utilized measurements of blood
variables to estimate the clinical activity of chronic bronchitis
in relation to clinical trials. In one study, we have followed
such patients with repeated measurements of serum levels of
lactoferrin, myeloperoxidase and lysozyme as markers of
neutrophil and monocyte/macrophage activity. We showed that these
patients have raised lysozyme levels, as signs of ongoing
activation of the macrophage population, irrespective of the
presence of infectious exacerbations. Lactoferrin and
myeloperoxidase levels, on the other hand, showed large
variations with peaks mostly coinciding with the infectious
exacerbations. In another study, we made repeated measurements
during a 6-months' period of a number of neutrophil activities.
These data showed increased activities with respect to migration
and oxidative metabolism during the period of increased numbers
of infectious exacerbations. All but one variable became normal
during periods of few infectious. Thus, the lucigenin-enhanced
chemiluminescence was subnormal during this period suggesting an
abnormality of neutrophil oxidative metabolism in patients with
chronic bronchitis. We conclude that the monitoring of markers of
inflammatory cell activity in serum may be useful as indicators
of the clinical activity of chronic bronchitis and that the
measurement of functional activities of the neutrophil is
dependent on seasonal variations in the exposure to infectious
agents in the community.

INTRODUCTION

One hallmark of patients with chronic bronchitis with or without obstructive lung disease is their recurrent infections of the airways (Sachs, 1981). The frequency of the infectious exacerbations vary considerably over the year, and exacerbations are generally more frequent during the autumn and winter seasons. In the monitoring of these patients for the purpose of drug intervention, this poses a problem, since the condition of a patient may vary spontaneously throughout the year, improvements occurring under certain periods irrespective of treatment. Also, the characterization and monitoring of these patients with different blood variables are likely to be influenced by seasonal variations, and results obtained during one period of the year may be very different from those obtained during another period. Few blood variables have been used to characterize patients with chronic bronchitis and to monitor the disease during pharmacological intervention. In particular, such studies have failed to considered the possible effects of infectious exacerbations and their seasonal variations. In this chapter, I will review some recent studies we have performed on patients with chronic bronchitis. In these studies, we focused on the activity of inflammatory cells such as neutrophils and monocytes, our hypothesis being that these cells are both involved in the pathogenesis of the disease and in the defence of the organism against invading microorganisms.

SERUM MEASUREMENTS OF INFLAMMATORY CELL MARKERS

In the first study, we followed a group of patients (n=34) with chronic bronchitis of stages 2 and 3 according to the definitions of the British Medical Research Council. Half of the patients served as a control group, the other being given a supposedly active therapy. The observation period started in October and ended in May the next year. The study was performed in collaboration with Dr. Ronald Dahl and his colleagues in Århus, Denmark (Venge et al., 1986). The patients monitored their symptoms in a number of respects, including their use of antibiotics and days of infections. In the control group, the accumulated number of infections per week was remarkably consistent throughout the whole observation period. Thus, on average, 4.5 of the individuals replied "yes" each week to the question "Have you had a cold?" and 3.5 each week to the question "Do you feel sick?", and these figures were identical during the entire observation period. Blood was drawn at regular intervals 5 times during the study for the counting of blood cells and differentials. Serum was prepared for the measurements of lysozyme as a marker of monocyte activity and lactoferrin and myeloperoxidase as markers of neutrophil activity. The results from the first and last week of observation are presented in Table I.

Table I. Blood-cell counts and serum levels of lysozyme, lactoferrin and myeloperoxidase in a group of patients with chronic bronchitis.

	Chronic Bronchitis	Controls	p-value
Lysozyme:			
October	2473±888 μg/l	1561±439 μg/l	<0.0001
May	2483±986 μg/l	− " −	<0.0001
Lactoferrin:			
October	754±560 μg/l	326±154 μg/l	<0.001
May	900±791 μg/l	− " −	<0.001
Myeloperoxidase:			
October	407±278 μg/l	201±171 μg/l	<0.05
May	303±212 μg/l	− " −	<0.05

The results are presented as means ±SD n=30 patients. The p-values indicate the differences as compared to a healthy reference population (n=90), in which no seasonal variations were observed. Student's t-test was used.

Leukocyte counts and differentials did not, on an average, differ from those of a healthy reference population at any time,

although some patients occasionally had transient leukocytosis
(leukocyte counts 7.74 ±2.80 and 6.87 ±1.57x10^9/l in October and
May, respectively, and neutrophil counts 64.2 ±12.6 and 59.7 ±9.5
%). The serum lysozyme levels were, however, highly and
significantly (p<0.0001) elevated at the start of the study and
remained unaltered during the whole period. The levels of
lactoferrin and myeloperoxidase were significantly elevated too,
(p<0.001 and p<0.05, respectively). These data suggest that both
macrophage/monocyte and neutrophil secretory activity is
increased in patients with chronic bronchitis. It is, however,
interesting that the individual variations of the neutrophil
markers were considerable in contrast to those of lysozyme, and
that there was no correlation between lysozyme and these two
other proteins. In some cases, we thus observed huge levels of
lactoferrin and myeloperoxidase but almost normal lysozyme levels
and vice versa. The consistency of the serum lysozyme levels was
reflected by the fact that the levels obtained at the start of
the study correlated significantly (p<0.001) to the succeeding
levels, linear correlation coefficients ranging from 0.83 to
0.89. This was contrasted by the lactoferrin and myeloperoxidase levels, which showed no such correlations. Our conclusions from these data are that monocyte/macrophage activity
is raised in patients with chronic bronchitis, but that this
increment is unaffected by the infectious exacerbations, whereas
neutrophil activity is raised occasionally, but mainly in
connection with infectious exacerbations. Unexpectedly, however,
we could not in this study discern any seasonal variations in the
number of infectious exacerbations or in blood variables.

MEASUREMENTS OF NEUTROPHIL FUNCTIONS

In the second study we measured a number of neutrophil functions
in a group of bronchitics. These patients were selected on the
basis of the same criteria as the ones stated above. They
included patients at stages 2 and 3 according to the definition

proposed by the British Medical Research Council and patients in whom the number of infectious exacerbations had been at least 2 during the two preceding winter seasons i.e. from October to April. The definition of an infectious exacerbation was the clinical indication of treating the infection with antibiotics. This study was carried out in collaboration with Dr. Sabina Rak and her colleagues at the Västerås county hospital in Sweden (Venge et al., 1989). The study comprised 48 patients 22 of whom were followed for 6 months, with monthly visits to the doctor. These patients were asked to keep diaries of their symptoms, making entries once a week according to a certain protocol. Once a month, blood was taken for the purpose of monitoring of blood-cell counts and differentials. Three times during the observation period, blood samples were drawn with a view to analyzing the functional activities of the neutrophils. The number of infectious exacerbations was significantly lower at the end of the observation period i.e. in April-May, than at the beginning of the study, i.e. in October-November (Table II).

Table II. Some blood variables and the number of infectious exacerbations in patients with chronic bronchitis and their seasonal variations

	Oct-Nov	April-May	p-value
Leukocyte count x 10^9/l	7.2 ± 2.0	6.8 ± 1.4	NS
Neutrophils %	58.3 ± 12.2	58.1 ± 7.6	NS
Eosinophils %	2.5 ± 1.0	3.0 ± 3.2	NS
Lymphocytes %	31.4 ± 11.3	31.2 ± 7.4	NS
Monocytes %	5.1 ± 2.7	5.7 ± 2.8	NS
Exacerbations	0.5 (0-3)	0 (0-3)	<0.05

Results are presented as means ±SD or as median and actual range (exacerbations). Statistical differences were calculated using paired T-test or Wilcoxon's sign rank test (exacerbations).

However, this reduction was not reflected by white-blood-cell numbers or differentials. Neutrophil migration was measured as spontaneous migration, i.e. random migration; as the chemotactic response towards a gradient of either the tripeptide FMLP or zymosan-activated serum, i.e. mainly C5-fragments, and as the chemo-kinetic response of the cells to normal and to the patient's own serum. Random migration and the chemotactic response to C5-fragments were significantly raised at the beginning of the observation period while being normal in April-May, whereas the other variables were similar to the controls during both periods (Table III). The phagocytic capacity of the neutrophils, as measured by the uptake of either IgG-coated or C3b-IgG-coated particles, was also normal during both periods. However, the opsonic activity of plasma - measured as the rate of opsonization of zymosan particles - was significantly raised in the patients during the first period but normal again in April-May. This probably reflects an increase in complement activity during the former period.

When we studied the capacity of the neutrophils to produce toxic oxygen metabolites such as H_2O_2 and O_2^- we found no alteration in the capacity to produce O_2^-, as measured by means of lucigenin-enhanced chemiluminescence, during the first period, but there was a significant reduction in this capacity during April-May. However, when we measured production of oxygen metabolites by means of luminol-enhanced chemiluminescence we found that it was raised during the first period but normal at the end of the period. Finally, lucigenin-enhanced chemi-luminescence of whole blood, which presumably chiefly reflects monocyte activity (Trulson et al., 1989), was significantly raised during the first period but normalized at the end of the study.

On the basis of these data, we concluded that all except one variable were normalized during a period of significantly fewer infections, and that the increased activities in several neutrophil functions are probably the outcome of ongoing sub-clinical infections (Pauksens et al., 1989; Pauksens & Venge, to

be published) rather than the results of specific abnormalities
found in patients with chronic bronchitis.

Table III. Some neutrophil functions in a group of patients
with chronic bronchitis and their seasonal variations.

	Chronic Bronchitis	Controls	p-value
Random migration:			
Oct-Nov	22±3 μm/h	19±4 μm/h	<0.01
April-May	18±3 μm/h***	- " -	NS
Chemotaxis towards zymosan-act. serum:			
Oct-Nov	107±20 μm/h	85±15 μm/h	<0.001
April-May	91±19 μm/h**	- " -	NS
Opsonic activity:			
Oct-Nov	2.3±0.91 min	3.7±1.8 min	<0.001
April-May	4.3±1.75 min***	- " -	NS
Luminol-enhanced CL, isolated PMN:			
Oct-Nov	61293±17027 RLU	46400±17500RLU	<0.001
April-May	51857±13661 RLU	- " -	NS
Lucigenin-enhanced CL, isolated PMN:			
Oct-Nov	11352±3657 RLU	12600±5100 RLU	NS
April-May	7767±2297 RLU***	- " -	<0.001
Luminol-enhanced CL whole-blood:			
Oct-Nov	703±420 RLU	397±187 RLU	<0.001
April-May	378±160 RLU**	- " -	NS
Lucigenin-enhanced CL, whole blood:			
Oct-Nov	566±422 RLU	343±144 RLU	<0.01
April-May	330±119 RLU*	- " -	NS

Results are expressed as means ±SD. p-values indicate the
differences as compared to a healthy reference population.
that was collected in parallel to the patients. In the
reference population, no seasonal variations were observed.
Differences between Oct-Nov and April-May are indicated by *,
, and * (p<0.05, 0.01, and 0.001, respectively). CL =
Chemiluminescence, RLU = Relative light units.

We also concluded that the only variable that was actually significantly reduced during the period of few infections, i.e. the capacity of the neutrophils to produce O_2^- may represent a true abnormality on the part of the patients and may in fact add to the predisposition of these patients to suffer recurrent bacterial infections. In this study, we thus saw a spontaneous clinical improvement which was associated with seasonal variation in the activities of the neutrophils. This study, therefore, clearly demonstrates the problems you may encounter when wishing to design a study of the efficacy of any drug in chronic bronchitis. The only feasible way to do this seems to be the study of parallel groups.

CONCLUSION: Our overall conclusion as to the monitoring of chronic bronchitis by means of blood samples is that no well-documented variables have been described previously, which could be of any help in this respect. Our own studies, however, have suggested that the use of specific markers of inflammatory cell activities - such as lysozyme as a marker of monocytes/ macrophages, and lactoferrin and myeloperoxidase as markers of neutrophils - may be used for these purposes. Also, the monitoring of neutrophil functions may be of value; but this is difficult to accomplish without immediate access to a specialized laboratory. Seasonal variations in several of these variables occur and have to be considered as well.

DISCUSSION

Stockley. As you know we have studied patients with clearly defined emphysema and shown that their neutrophils demonstrate an increased chemotactic response and degranulation compared to control subjects. However, I cannot remember what time of year they were studied and your data suggests this might have been important.

I have three questions. Firstly, did you assess your control subjects on the same three occasions as the patients? Secondly, you call them chronic bronchitis patients, can you define them more clearly? Finally were the patients on any therapy that could alter neutrophil function such as macrolide antibiotics or steroid therapy?

Venge. The answer to your first question is yes we did, but as there were no differences between the seasons, the results were pooled for the controls. The patients were classified according the criteria of the British Medical Research Council (1965). Two patients had inhaled GCS, but I have no details on these patients.

Brattsand. Do you believe that the seasonal variation is primary or secondary to infection periods?

Venge. I believe that most of what we see is secondary to infection periods although we were careful not to sample from patients with clinically overt disease.

Brattsand. The occurrence of this seasonal variation makes a risk that unethical clinicians and pharmaceutical industries can design uncontrolled clinical trials so that they can more easily reach the results they want.

Venge. Yes, I agree.

Hogg. Subjects who smoke have higher circulating WBC counts. Were there any differences in the level of smoking between your groups or any difference in the WBC counts?

Venge. No.

Brattsand. From your presentation I find the lucigenin findings the most deviating property of the bronchitic, because this

parameter was not normalized even during the spring period, when
they were without exacerbation. Therefore, I suggest this
parameter to be central in forthcoming studies.

Venge. It is true that this variable was the only one, that was
significantly reduced as compared to normals. This could be a
reflection of the fact that patients with chronic bronchitis and
recurrent infections (exacerbations) have really a defect in
neutrophil function that predisposes them to these infections.

Hargreave. What is known about these parameters in asthma?

Venge. We have so far measured only the chemokinetic and
chemotactic activity of neutrophils in asthma. These activities
are basically normal in contrast to the activity of the
eosinophils which is primed to an enhanced responsiveness to
chemokinetic and chemotactic factors.

Chung. We also found that in asthmatic patients there is
enhancement of lucigenin-dependent chemiluminescence induced by
phorbol myristate acetate and platelet activating factor in
circulating eosinophils, but not in circulating neutrophils.

Stockley. I could comment that we have also looked at patients
with bronchiectasis who have a continued infection. The
neutrophils from these patients were not more sensitive to a
chemotactic stimulus compared to healthy subjects. This was
clearly different from the patients with emphysema.

REFERENCES

Pauksens, K., Sjölin, J., and Venge, P. (1989) Scand. J. Infect.
    Dis. 21, 277-284.
Sachs, F.L. (1981) Clinics in Chest Medicine, 2, 79-89.
Trulson, A., Nilsson, S., and Venge, P. (1989) Am. J. Clin.
    Pathol. 91, 441-445.
Venge, P., Dahl, R., Håkansson, L., Hällgren, R., Lindblad, G.,

and Pedersen, B. (1986) Abstract presented at the 4th
International symposium on infections in the
immunocompromised host. 137.
Venge, P., Rak, S., Steinholtz, L., Håkansson, L., and
Lindblad, G. (1989) Submitted for publication.

9) SEASONAL VARIATION IN THE PHAGOCYTIC ACTIVITY AND ARACHIDONIC-ACID METABOLISM OF HUMAN BLOOD MONOCYTES IN HEALTHY NON-SMOKERS, SMOKERS AND CHRONIC BRONCHITICS.

Margareta Linden[1], M. Larsson[2], T. Prellner[3], and R. Brattsand[1].

[1]Laboratory of Pharmacology, Research & Development Department, AB Draco, Box 34, S-221 00 Lund, Sweden. [2]Medical Department, AB Draco, Lund, Sweden. [3]Department of Infectious Diseases, Malmö General Hospital, S-221 00 Lund, Sweden.

SUMMARY: Peripheral blood monocytes are precursor cells to alveolar macrophages (AMs). Many studies have been performed with a view to assessing the differences, in respect of morphology and function, between the AMs of smokers and those of non-smokers. Disturbed host-defence activity of smokers' AMs is reflected by, for instance, decreased phagocytic activity and impaired arachidonic acid metabolism. However, very little attention has been paid to the question what effects cigarette smoking and chronic bronchitis may have on the function of the precursors of these cells - the blood monocytes. The collection of blood monocytes is much less laborious than the sampling of AMs. Therefore, it would be a great advance if the deteriorated host defence in chronic bronchitis could be detected and followed by studies of blood monocytes. However, a seasonal variation in monocyte function, discussed in this paper, may counteract the advantage inherent in repeated sampling. This seasonal variation in cellular host-defence mechanisms should be taken into account when designing longitudinal intervention trials in chronic bronchitis.

INTRODUCTION

Cigarette smoking is clearly related to chronic bronchitis (CB), a condition marked not only by an overproduction of bronchial secretions but also by disability due to recurrent bacterial and viral infections. The increased susceptibility to infections which is characteristic of chronic bronchitis may be a result of impaired defence mechanisms in the lung (Holt, 1987) as well as in the systemic compartment (Nielsen & Bonde, 1986; Fietta et al., 1988).

The alveolar macrophage (AM) plays a key role in defending the lung against inhaled particular matter and invading micro-organisms. Many studies have been performed in order to assess differences, with regard to morphology and functional parameters (for a review, see Holt, 1987) between the AMs of smokers and those of non-smokers. Cigarette smoking may decrease the phagocytic activity of AMs (Martin & Warr, 1977; Fischer et al., 1982; Linden et al., 1988). Smoking also appears to impair the metabolism of arachidonic acid, because the secretion of prostaglandin E_2 (PGE_2), $PGF_{2\alpha}$, 5-HETE and leukotriene B_4 (LTB_4) are all significantly reduced, particularly after stimulation (Laviolette et al., 1981; 1986; Wieslander et al., 1987). However, other aspects of AM activity, e.g. the production of oxygen radicals, may be less influenced or even stimulated by smoking (Bergstrand, 1990).

The majority of AMs are derived from circulating blood monocytes (Blusse et al., 1983). However, relatively little attention has been paid to the question what effects cigarette smoking and chronic bronchitis may have on the function of these precursor cells to AMs. Nielsen (1985) and Nielsen & Bonde (1986) reported an impaired phagocytic activity in the blood monocytes of healthy smokers and in those of patients with chronic bronchitis. The metabolism of arachidonic acid in the monocytes of smokers and chronic bronchitics has not been studied to an appreciable extent.

The collection of alveolar macrophages is a much more

laborious procedure than the sampling and preparation of blood monocytes. Therefore, from a practical point of view, it would be a big advance (facilitating repeated sampling) in longitudinal inter-vention studies if the deteriorated host defence of chronic bronchitis could be detected and followed via functional studies of blood monocytes instead of alveolar macrophages. However, the advantage of repeated sampling might be counteracted by a poten-tial seasonal variation in the cellular host-defence mechanisms. These issues have not been carefully investigated, in spite of the great importance that the answers would have when designing optimal longitudinal intervention trials in chronic bronchitis.

To elucidate these questions, three blood-monocyte functions were determined in vitro as parameters of systemic host-defence activity in 12 healthy non-smokers (mean age 51 ± 2 years, mean ± SEM), in 12 healthy smokers (48 ± 3 years) and in 12 chronic bronchitics (51 ± 3 years) (Linden et al., 1988a). In the last group all but one were smokers, and all had recurrent infections. All subjects were free of clinical infections at least 2 weeks prior to blood sampling. In order to investigate whether the well-known seasonal variation in CB symptoms might be related to alterations in monocyte func-tion, all subjects were tested during three seasons (May-June, October-November, February).

PHAGOCYTOSIS

The phagocytic activity of the blood monocytes was determined in an in vitro assay (Linden et al., 1988b), based on the uptake of opsonized yeast particles. In all the three groups that were studied, there was a seasonal variation in the percentage of ingesting cells (Fig. 1). However, no such variation was noted for the number of phagocytosed particles per active cell. In all three groups, the percentage of ingesting monocytes was at least 10 % lower (P<0.01) in May-June than in February (Fig. 1). In the two smoking groups, the value pertaining to October-November ranked in between the phagocytosis values referring to the other two periods.

A negative influence on monocyte phagocytosis exercised by smoking and by chronic bronchitis was demonstrated when the subjects were compared during the May-June period (Fig. 1). The mean frequency of ingesting monocytes was then ~15 % lower (P<0.01) among the bronchitics than among the non-smoking controls. However, no such negative influence could be observed during the other two seasons.

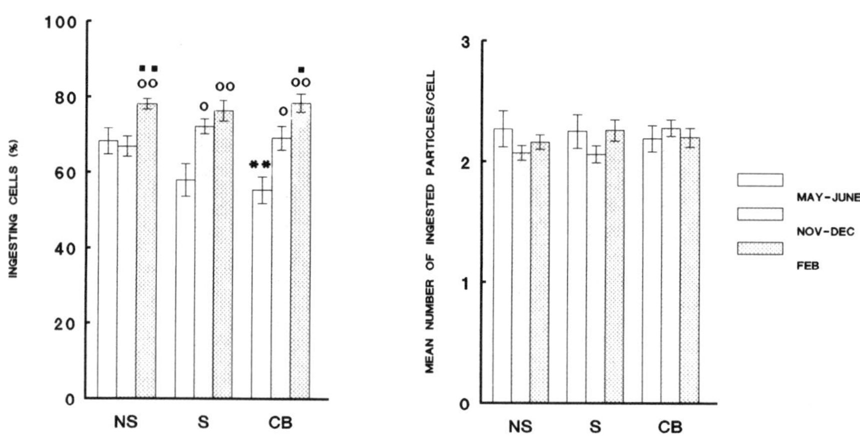

Figure 1. Blood monocytes were separated by means of density centrifugation on Mono-Poly Resolving Medium (Flow Lab) and, after repeated washings, resuspended in RPMI 1640 (Flow), supplemented with 5 % fetal calf serum and gentamycin (50 μl/ml). The phagocytosis of fluorescein-labelled yeast particles by the adhered monocytes was determined according to a modification (Linden et al., 1988b) of the method described by Hed (1977). The results are expressed as mean ± SEM. Comparisons between groups were performed with the Mann-Whitney U test for unpaired data. Intra-group comparisons between seasons were performed using Wilcoxon's signed rank test for paired observations.
NS: non-smokers, S: smokers, CB: chronic bronchitics
*: p<0.05, **: p<0.01 compared with non-smokers
o: p<0.05, oo: p<0.01 "   "   May-June
■: p<0.05, ■■: p<0.01 "   "   Nov-Dec

THE SECRETION OF ARACHIDONIC-ACID METABOLITES

A stimulation of the arachidonic-acid metabolism is held to be one important part of the host-defence activity of macrophages/ monocytes (Holt, 1987). Such stimulation will reinforce the local inflammation by releasing mediators such as prostaglandin E_2 (inducing vasodilatation); leukotrienes C_4 and D_4, thromboxanes and PAF (enhancing vascular leakiness); leukotriene B_4 and PAF (chemotactic for leukocytes). The contention that this release of pro-inflammatory mediators is important to a proper host-defence reactivity is supported by the experimental and clinical knowledge that intense anti-inflammatory treatment with glucocorticoids, which will block (among other things) the arachidonic-acid metabolism, leads to an enhanced risk of infections spreading.

Against this background, the ability of blood monocytes to release PGE_2 and LTB_4 was investigated as a potential part of systemic host-defence function. The results pertaining to the stimulated release of PGE_2 are shown in Fig. 2. A marked seasonal variation was noted in all three groups, the trend being the same as the one described above, with a much higher monocyte activity during autumn-winter ($P<0.05-0.01$) than during spring. The only exception was the October-November value of the smokers, where the elevation from spring to autumn did not reach statistical significance.

When compared to the healthy non-smokers, the smokers ($P<0.01$) as well as the bronchitics ($P<0.05$) had a reduced PGE_2 secretion during the May-June period (Fig 2). A similar difference as compared to the non-smokers existed among the smokers ($P<0.01$) during October-November, too. However, in February, when secretion was high in all groups, no significant differences between the groups could be demonstrated.

The secretion of LTB_4 varied in a partly different manner (Fig. 3). Secretion rose from May-June to October-November, but that elevation was significant ($P<0.01$) among the healthy non-smokers only. In the latter group, the LTB_4 secretion returned to the

preceding spring level in February. In the other two groups,
seasonal variation was less marked, a slight but non-significant
rising trend being observable from spring by way of autumn to
winter.

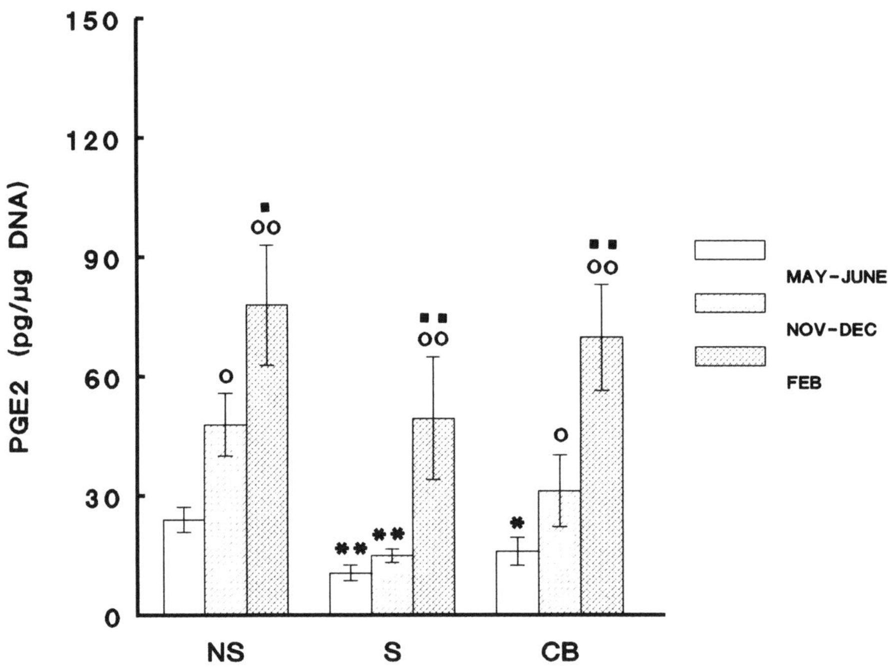

Figure 2. Blood monocytes (97-99 % purity and 98±1
viability) were separated by means of density centrifugation
(Monopoly Resolving Medium, Flow Lab), adherence overnight in
tissue-culture multidishes (Nunc, Denmark). After stimulation for
90 min with human serum opsonized zymosan, the culture medium was
analyzed for PGE_2 by means of radioimmunoassay (New England
Nuclear, Sweden). The PGE_2 content was related to the DNA-content
(Labarca and Paigen 1980) of the cultures. The results are
expressed as mean ± SEM. Comparisons between groups were
performed with the Mann-Whitney U test for unpaired data. Intra-
group comparisons between seasons were performed using Wilcoxon's
signed rank test for paired observations.
NS: non-smokers, S: smokers, CB: chronic bronchitics
*: p<0.05, **: p<0.01 compared with non-smokers
o: p<0.05, oo: p<0.01 "   "   May-June
■: p<0.05, ■■: p<0.01 "   "   Nov-Dec

When compared within the seasonal periods, both smokers and bronchitics had a significantly (P<0.05-0.01) reduced LTB$_4$ secretion during October-November (Fig. 3). No such difference was reached during the other two periods.

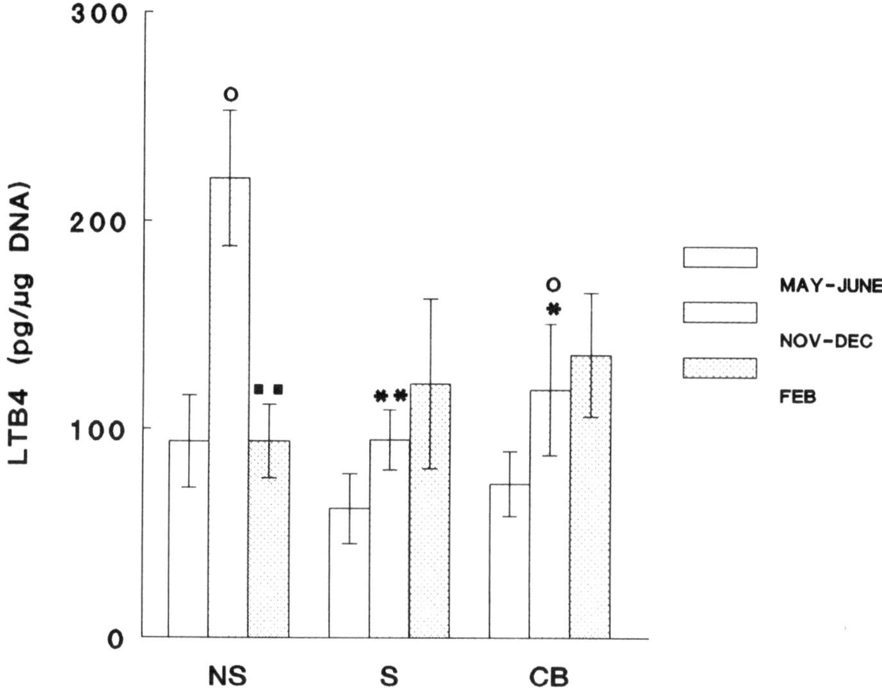

Figure 3. Blood monocytes were separated and challenged as described in Fig. 2. The LTB$_4$-content of the medium was determined by means of RIA (New England Nuclear, Sweden) and related to the DNA content as described in Fig. 2. The results are expressed as mean ± SEM. Comparisons between groups were performed with the Mann-Whitney U test for unpaired data. Intra-group comparisons between seasons were performed using Wilcoxon's signed rank test for paired observations.
NS: non-smokers, S: smokers, CB: chronic bronchitics
*: p<0.05, **: p<0.01 compared with non-smokers
o: p<0.05, oo: p<0.01 "   "   May-June
■: p<0.05, ■■: p<0.01 "   "   Nov-Dec

SUPPORT FOR THE BELIEF THAT SEASONAL VARIATION
AFFECTS MONOCYTE ACTIVITY

A similar trend was observed with regard to most of the monocyte activities that were studied: cells collected during autumn were more active than those sampled in spring. In respect of phagocytosis and the secretion of PGE_2 this enhanced activity also persisted regarding cells collected in February. A similar tendency towards higher cellular activity during autumn than in spring has been described in respect of the blood neutrophils of bronchitics (Venge 1990 - preceding chapter). Although the current trial was only implemented during a ten-month period, the changing activity is interpreted as a seasonal variation. The reasons for this type of seasonal variation are not well known. One potential reason might be a general priming of the immune system during autumn and winter due to the higher prevalence of respiratory infections in the community during these periods. Furthermore, hormonal factors influencing the immune system may change during the dark seasons as compared with spring and summer. There is no support for the belief that a seasonal variation affects the monocyte numbers of bronchitics (Venge, 1990). Regarding external climate factors, it has been demonstrated, by Chavance and colleagues (1988), that periods with cold weather correlate to temporary rises in basophil counts. Also, the B cell/T cell ratio in normal human peripheral blood is increased during the coldest months (Bratescu & Teodorescu, 1981).

THE PATHOPHYSIOLOGY OF CHRONIC BRONCHITIS IN RELATION
TO MACROPHAGE/ MONOCYTE ACTIVITY

As was stated in the introduction, cigarette smoking and chronic bronchitis impair phagocytosis (Martin & Warr 1977; Fischer et al., 1982; Linden et al., 1988b) as well as some of the secretory activities (Laviolette et al., 1981, 1986; Wieslander et al.,

1988) of alveolar macrophages. This impaired phagocyte function within the human lung may contribute to the immunosuppression induced by smoking in the immune-mediated lung diseases sarcoidosis and extrinsic allergic alveolitis (Sharma, 1985). Considering the central role played by the alveolar macrophage in connection with the initiation, and the exertion, of host-defence action in the lung, it is tempting to speculate that the smoke-induced suppression of the macrophage function might even facilitate - directly or indirectly - the respiratory infections possibly underlying bronchitic exacerbations.

The current study supports other findings (Nielsen, 1985; Nielsen & Bonde 1986; Fietta et al., 1988; Venge, 1990) demonstrating that smoking and bronchitis impair the function of the precursors of alveolar macrophages, the blood monocytes. Thus, smoking may affect host-defence activity in the systemic compartment, too. Due to the feasibility of monocyte sampling this opens up novel possibilities for longitudinal studies on the smoke-induced modulation of the phagocyte function. Our study proposes that the impaired function is best elucidated in spring. It also suggests that the absolute level of monocyte activity does not directly relate to respiratory morbidity; if it did, bronchitics should suffer their highest rate of exacerbations during spring and not - which is actually the case - during autumn and winter. However, the results may be taken to indicate that the basic monocyte defect is least influenced by other priming events in spring, as a result of - for instance - a reduced number of respiratory infections in the community, or hormonal priming, at that time. The results obtained during the two following seasons show that bronchitics can enhance their monocyte activity by some, still unknown, mechanism. However, the LTB$_4$ secretion was still significantly reduced during the autumn in the bronchitic group. The increments may be insufficient to compensate for all the encumbrances induced by smoking and/or exacerbations. In order to elucidate the importance of a depressed phagocyte function, more investigations are required, dealing with the effect of immunostimulation on monocyte/macro-

phage activity in relation to its impact on the exacerbation
rate.

SEASONAL VARIATION – ITS IMPORTANCE WHEN DESIGNING
INTERVENTION STUDIES

Thus, besides the well-known seasonal variation in the symptoms
of chronic bronchitis, there is now growing evidence in favour
of the view that seasonal variation may also affect blood-
phagocyte functions (monocytes – this report; neutrophils –
Venge, 1990). Whether a similar variation also occurs in
alveolar-macrophage functions is still unknown.

With this knowledge in mind, controlled clinical trials based
on symptoms (e.g. exacerbation rate) as well as on cellular-
biochemical parameters should be organized as comparisons between
parallel groups rather than as cross-over comparisons involving
different seasons for the active and placebo periods. The
awareness of seasonal variation should also operate when
reevaluating earlier cross-over trials.

DISCUSSION

Hogg. Do monocytes that have adhered to glass behave differently
than those that do not?

Margareta Linden. I have no data on monocytes. However, I have
studied alveolar macrophages (AMs) from guinea pig. AMs were
purified by centrifugal elutriation and cultured in suspension or
they were separated by adherence to plastic surface. AMs cultured
in suspension released less LTB_4, than did AMs cultured in
monolayers. Thus, the response of adherent cells was different
from that of suspended cells.

Nielsen. 1. Have you tried phagocytosis assay in suspension?

2. What is the exact number of effector cells (macrophages) on the glass slides?
3. The percentage of monocytes in mononuclear cell suspensions may vary greatly, do you adjust the number of monocytes?

Margareta Linden. 1. No
2. One million mononuclear cells are seeded in each test. However, we don't know how many of these that will adhere to the microscope slide.
3. Of the cells adhering to the glass slide, 97-99 % are monocytes.

Stockley. I have a technical comment. It has been conventional to purify monocytes by an adherence step. This clearly separates a minor proportion of cells. Of the remainder a proportion will adhere in the presence of endotoxin and the rest will not. These 3 populations behave very differently in terms of phagocytosis, superoxide production and protein production as well as "macrophage" surface markers. Ficoll invariably contains endotoxin and this will also affect the results. Thus, until the function of these subsets of monocytes is understood, it is wisest to study them all. In addition, separation techniques should avoid endotoxin contaminated reagents.

Margareta Linden. The same batch of Ficoll-Hypaque gradient was used throughout the whole study. This reduces the problem with endotoxin. About 50 % of seeded monocytes will adhere to the plastic surface. Thus, we are studying a subpopulation of monocytes.

Eriksson. Do you think that the significant but relatively small differences between healthy volunteers and chronic bronchitics can be important as markers for inflammation in the light of the great seasonal variation in the healthy volunteers?

Margareta Linden. My answer is yes. However, to study the differences a parallel group design is to be preferred before cross-over. A placebo group should be included to reduce the importance of seasonal variation.

REFERENCES

Bergstrand H. This volume.
Blusse Van Oud Alblas, A., Van Der Linden-Schrever, B., and Van Furth, R. (1983) Am. Rev. Respir. Dis. 128, 276-281.
Bratescu, A., and Teodorescu, M. (1981) J. Allergy Clin. Immunol. 68, 273-280.
Chavance, M., Herberth, B., and Kauffmann, F. (1988) Int. Arch. Allergy Appl. Immunol. 86, 462-464.
Fietta, A., Bersani, C., De Rose, V., Grassi, F.A., Mangiarotti, P., Uccelli, M., and Grassi C. (1988) Respiration 53, 37-43.
Fisher, G.L., McNeil, K.L., Finch, G.L., Wilson, F.D., and Golde, D.W. (1982) J. Reticuloendoth. Soc. 32, 311-321.
Holt, P.G. (1987) Thorax 42, 241-249.
Hed, J. (1977) FEMS Microbiol. Lett. 1, 357-361.
Labarca, C., and Paigen, K. (1980) Anal. Biochem. 102, 344-352.
Laviolette, M., Chang, J., and Newcombe, D.S. (1981) Am. Rev. Respir. Dis. 124, 397-401.
Laviolette, M., Coulombe, R., Picxard, S., Braquet, P., and Borgeat, P. (1986) J. Clin. Invest. 77, 54-60.
Linden, M., Anderson, E., Prellner, T., and Brattsand, R. (1988a) Second International Conf. on Leukotrienes & Prostanoids in Health & Disease, Jerusalem.
Linden M., Wieslander, E., Eklund, A., Larsson, K., and Brattsand, R. (1988b) Eur. Respir. J. 1, 645-650.
Martin, R.R., and Warr, G.A. (1977) Hosp. Practice 86, 97-104.
Nielsen, H. (1985) Eur. J. Respir. Dis. 66, 327-332.
Nielsen, H., and Bonde, J. (1986) Eur. J. Respir. Dis. 68, 200-206.
Sharma, P.O. (1985) Sarcoidosis 2, 9-11.
Venge, P. (1990) This volume.
Wieslander, E., Linden, M., Håkansson, L., Eklund, A., Blaschke, E., Brattsand, R., and Venge, P. (1987) Eur. J. Respir. Dis. 71, 263-272.

10)   A CRITICAL VIEW ON LAVAGE SAMPLING TECHNIQUES

Birgitta Schmekel

Department of Lung Medicine, University Hospital, Lund, and
Department of Explorative Clinical Research, AB Draco, Box 34,
S-211 00 Lund, Sweden.

SUMMARY: The constituents of the liquid aspirated in bronchoalveolar lavage are determined by the distribution of the fluid
within the bronchial tree, the diffusion through membranes and
the dilution by body fluids. Small volume lavages, sample cells,
and soluble constituents from the surfaces of the proximal
bronchial tree, and usually contain fewer cells than large volume
bronchoalveolar lavages.

INTRODUCTION

The sampling of airway lining cells and fluid-phase constituents
by means of bronchoalveolar lavage (BAL) is a well-established
research instrument. Although BAL has been performed for many
years, little has been done to standardize the technique. A
number of factors may contribute to the composition of fluid-
phase constituents in lavage fluid, and some of them will be
reviewed in the present paper.

Sequential division of the human airways results in approximately twenty-two to twenty-five generations of airways. Columnar
ciliated epithelial cells and submucosal glands are located in
the luminal part of the airways, from the trachea to the terminal

bronchi. The most consistent abnormal biopsy findings in chronic bronchitis are found in the bronchial and the bronchiolar regions. The selective sampling of material from these parts of the airways would therefore be preferential in studies on chronic bronchitis.

METHODOLOGICAL ASPECTS

<u>Distribution of injected lavage fluid</u>: The anatomical distribution of injected lavage fluid has been studied by means of digital subtraction-radiography (Kelly et al., 1987). It was shown that the first of sequentially injected 60 ml aliquots stayed close to the bronchoscope, sampling fluid in the proximal airways. In contrast, the following two aliquots sampled fluid from both distal airways and alveoli. Also, other indices of airway sampling by the first injected aliquot have been presented (Martin et al., 1985). In agreement with those findings, we found significantly higher proportions of ciliated epithelial cells ($p<0.05$) as well as of neutrophils ($p<0.001$) in the first of four sequential 50 ml aliquots (Fig. 1a + 1b), which suggested a sampling area corresponding to proximal airways in the first aspirated aliquot (unpublished observations).

It has been shown that proportionately lower volumes are recovered from subjects with obstructive lung diseases (Martin et al., 1985) and from healthy subjects lavaged in the lower as compared to the middle lobe (Pingleton et al., 1983). Four aliquots of 50 ml warm saline were sequentially infused in the right middle lobe and gently aspirated with a standardized suction pressure in five healthy smokers and seven healthy non-smokers (Fig. 1c). The recovery volumes tended to increase within the series in the non-smokers, in contrast to findings in smokers. The volumes of the fourth aliquots aspirated were significantly lower in smokers as compared to non-smokers ($p<0.01$). Differences in bronchial wall compliance in smokers and nonsmokers may therefore interact with the proportion of the infused fluid volume recovered by aspiration.

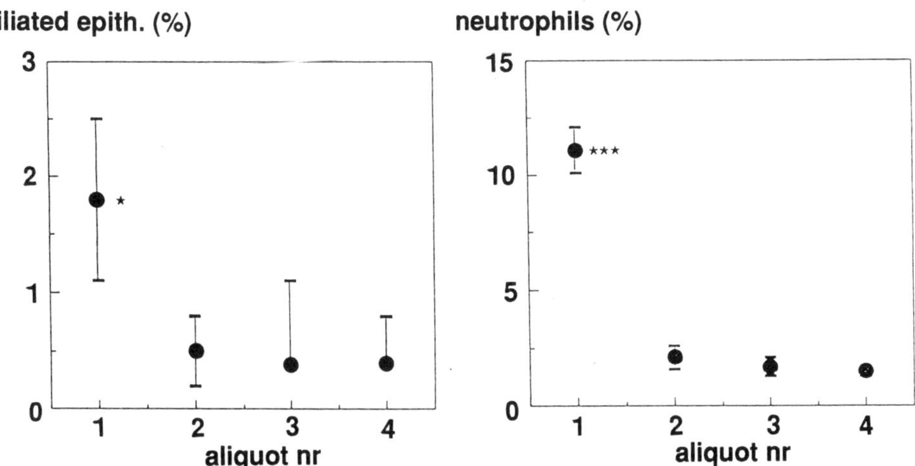

Figure 1a & 1b. The recovery of ciliated epithelial cells (a) or neutrophil cells (b) in sequential lavage (4 x 50 ml), performed on seven healthy non-smokers. The cell number is expressed as a percentage of the total cell-number, mean and SEM are given, and the significant difference between the first and second aliquot is indicated by * = p<0.05 or *** = p<0.001.

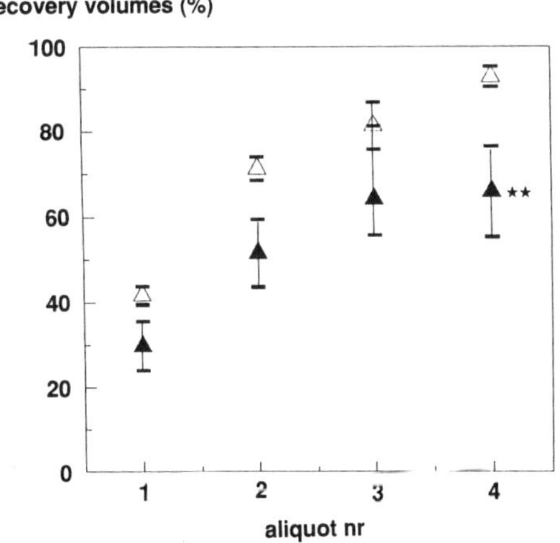

Figure 1c. The recovery volumes in sequential lavage (4x50 ml) performed on seven healthy non-smokers (open triangles) and five healthy smokers (closed triangles). Mean volumes and SEM are indicated. Significant differences in volumes recovered from non-smokers and smokers are indicated for each aliquot number. ** = p<0.01.

                                                           B. Schmekel

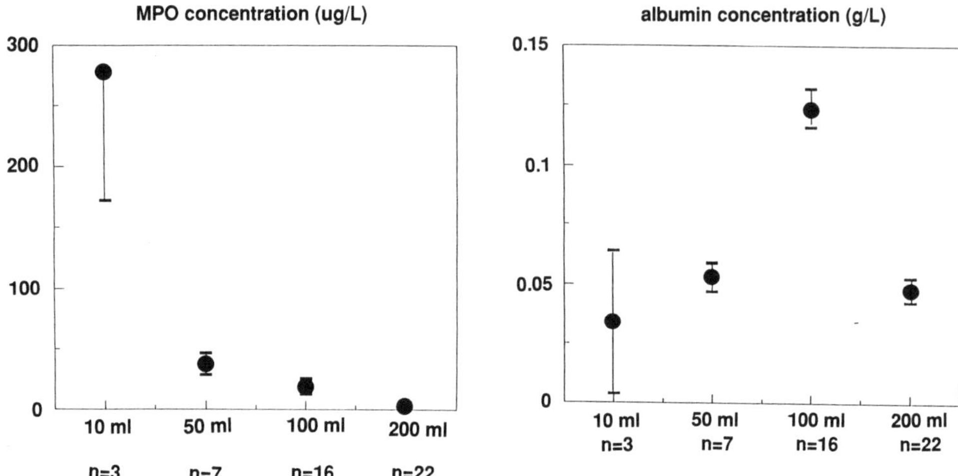

Figure 2a & 2b. The concentration of myeloperoxidase (MPO) (a) or albumin (b) in BAL fluid, when various volumes were infused. Mean values and SEM are indicated.

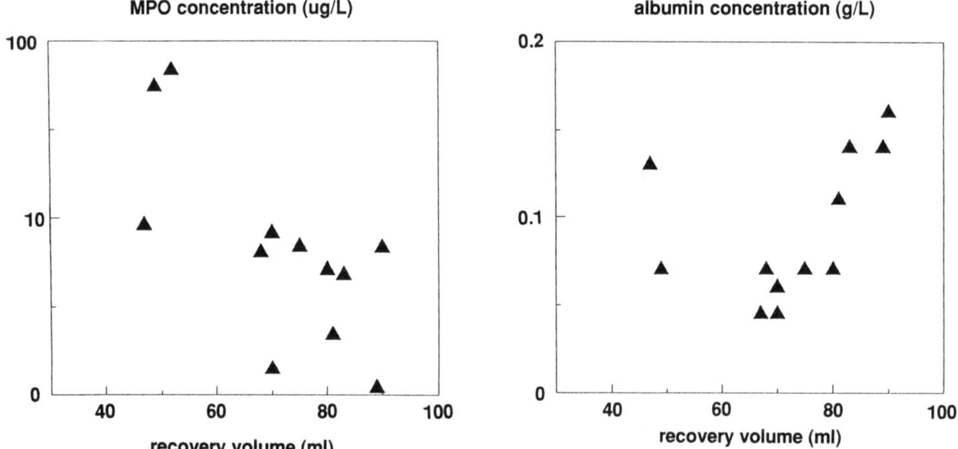

Figure 2c & 2d. BAL concentration of myeloperoxidase (MPO) (c) or albumin (d) versus recovery volumes of 24 healthy subjects who underwent to BAL in the right middle lobe. Values for the first (bronchial) aliquot are not given; the second and third pooled aliquots were used for measurements of the proteins. The recovery volumes were significantly correlated to the MPO concentrations (r=0.763, p=0.002) but not to the albumin concentrations (r=-0.02, p>0.05).

Quantitation of soluble substances: Attempts to quantitate soluble substances in BAL fluid have elicited considerable controversy. Because the retrieval of epithelial lining fluid necessitates the infusion of saline, the epithelial lining fluid is diluted by a variable amount of saline solution. The infusion and aspiration of various lavage volumes may yield various concentrations of a certain substance (Myeloperoxidase, Fig. 2a), while the recovery of another substance may show a completely different concentration pattern (Albumin, Fig. 2b). In addition, the recovery of these substances may (Fig. 2c) or may not (Fig. 2d) depend on the volumes aspirated, which may in turn be determined by the bronchial-wall compliance. The distribution of the lowest volumes of aspirated lavage fluid in the proximal airways (Kelly et al., 1987), therefore suggests myeloperoxidase to be located mainly in proximal airways. These findings are in agreement with the finding of higher proportions of neutrophils in the first aspirated aliquot (Fig. 1b). Higher concentrations of albumin in lavage fluids with larger volumes, would then suggest higher concentrations of this protein in the peripheral parts of the airways. Simple dilution models appear not to govern the recoveries of soluble substances as previously shown by others (Davis et al., 1982; Merrill et al., 1982; Lam et al., 1985). The composition of the lavage aspirates appears to be influenced by the distribution of the fluid within the bronchial tree, which in turn may be determined by the bronchial wall compliance. The dilution by body fluids and the diffusion of saline from the airways during the lavage may also interfere with the composition of the aspirated fluids.

Therefore, a presentation of the total amount of recovered molecules or an expression of the concentration of a given molecule per unit of returned lavage fluid, may only be relevant in comparisons of soluble substances between groups of subjects when infused and aspirated volumes are comparable.

Attempts to circumvent the difficulties inherent in estimations of local concentrations of soluble substances in epithelial lining fluid have been made, using external markers of dilution. Inulin and methylene blue (Baughman et al., 1983), 99mTc-colloid and tritiated water (Kelly et al., 1988) are examples of markers that have been employed for this purpose. The dilution of tritiated water in lavage fluid indicated a total fluid gain of around 44 % in a lavage study using 3 x 60 ml aliquots. The use of endogenous markers for the diffusion of fluid through membranes has also been reported (Rennard et al., 1986). The method of quantitation of urea in BAL as a means of determining the volume of epithelial lining fluid assumes that urea does not diffuse from plasma into the instilled saline during the lavage procedure. However, it has been shown that a significant amount of urea does diffuse into the instilled BAL fluid (Marcy et al., 1987). These findings are in agreement with findings in BAL fluid from 24 healthy subjects, lavaged in the right middle lobe. The fluid was aspirated 2 to 5.2 minutes after the infusion of saline, and there was a significant correlation between the BAL concentration of urea and the maximal dwell time of lavage fluid (r=0.717, p<0.001) (unpublished observations).

In a study by Kelly et al. (1988), urea and tritiated water were used as endogenous markers, and it was calculated that resident fluid contributed less than 2 % of the total aspirated volume. It was concluded that "large volumes of fluid do appear to cross the alveolar membrane in both directions during lavage, the net result being an influx of fluid from the circulation into the lung."

<u>Sequential recovery of soluble substances</u>: The soluble substances recovered from the airways by way of lavage may be studied by means of the sequential infusion and aspiration of a series of 10 ml lavages. Sixteen aliquots of 10 ml of saline were sequentially injected and aspirated (Schmekel & Venge, 1990). The total contents of myeloperoxidase (MPO), eosinophil cationic protein (ECP), albumin and urea were calculated, and the accumulated total contents were plotted versus the serial aliquot numbers. The accumulated MPO contents reached a plateau after five aspirated aliquots, ECP after 7-8 aliquots, and albumin after 10-

12 aliquots. These findings are consistent with the conception of sequential emptying of a bronchial compartment. This compartment would then be defined as a relatively small area of proximal bronchial mucosal membrane, since it appears to be emptied by a limited number of lavage aliquots. MPO is a marker of neutrophil activity in BAL (Schmekel et al., 1990), and the observation that the first ("bronchial") aliquot of the lavage contains more neutrophils than the following ("bronchoalveolar") aliquots, is compatible with the conception of a relatively small compartment close to the tip of the bronchoscope, sampled by the first 50 ml of lavage fluid, containing neutrophils and their secretory products. These findings are supported by the results illustrated in Fig. 1b and 2a. The ECP content of the bronchial compartment seems to be emptied slightly after that of MPO, a finding which agrees with the observation that eosinophil cells in lavage fluid do not significantly decrease after the first 50 ml aliquot, but rather tends to fluctuate or slowly decrease throughout a sequential series (unpublished observations). The variability of the albumin content was great in this series, presumably due to technical difficulties in measuring the low concentrations in the fluids. The accumulated contents of urea did not reach a plateau even after 16 aspirated aliquots, but showed a successive increase throughout the series. The findings of continuously increasing accumulated total contents of urea, agrees with the conception that urea diffuses freely through membranes and is continuously accumulated in the lavage during the lavage process. It was previously suggested that lavage fluid retention times longer than one minute may interfere with the recovery of urea in BAL (Marcy et al., 1987). The dwell times of these small aliquots of lavage fluids were all less than 30 seconds, but since only around 50 % of the fluid was recovered in each aliquot, parts of the injected fluid may have longer retention times, which may in turn have influenced the concentration of urea towards the end of the sequence.

Reproducibility: The inter- and intrapersonal variability of soluble substances in lavage has not been extensively studied. In one study the concordance of secretory components and other proteins was reported to be good (Merrill et al., 1980). The lavage of different areas of the lung, and separate analyses of the samples, would provide an internal control of reproducibility.

Clinical relevance: The clinical relevance of BAL, as well as the diagnostic ability of the lavage method when it comes to predicting clinical course or therapeutic effect, has caused considerable controversy. The limitations of the method are obvious - lavage only samples the airspaces of a subsegment of a lobe and may not be representative of the whole lung nor of the intramural or parenchymal tissue. It seems, however, apparent that events in the proximal airways are satisfactorily reflected by small-volume lavages. In addition, lavage samples may reflect diseases occurring in the airspace more directly than blood and may therefore supply a better information than a remote specimen such as blood. The value of lavage monitoring with a view to predicting clinical outcome, in patients with chronic bronchitis could be considerable, provided the appropriate markers in lavage fluid are identified.

CONCLUSION: Diffusion through lung membranes during the lavage procedure appears to be lower in the first aspirated (bronchial) aliquot than in the following (bronchoalveolar) aliquots (Kelly et al., 1988). As the bronchial washes contain too few cells for most cell-functional analyses, it appears that BAL studies of patients with bronchial diseases could preferentially be performed by way of measuring soluble substances in bronchial-lavage fluid. To collect bronchial washes, the infused volumes should be limited to 50 or 60 ml. Larger lavage volumes appear to collect cells and soluble substances from more peripheral parts of the lung and to contain more cells.

External markers, such as methylene blue, ^{99m}Tc-colloid, tritiated water or any other suitable marker, should be added to the lavage fluid for the purpose of estimating dilution. Alternatively, a series of sequential small lavages, performed in order to assess the total amounts of the fluid-phase constituents in the bronchial compartment, could be subjected to comparative analysis.

DISCUSSION

Stockley. As you have shown there are differences of opinion on how to perform a lavage and what it samples. There was a meeting in Maryland in 1984 to discuss this but no consensus of opinion was reached. Perhaps it doesn't matter as long as the method is constant for the patients before and after intervention. The data you have shown suggests that most of the protein is recovered by the first 100 ml and most of the myeloperoxidase after 50 ml. This suggests that 0-50 ml is reasonable for a bronchial lavage and 50 to 100 ml for a bronchoalveolar lavage. Indeed most workers believe that 100 ml is the minimum volume required for BAL.

Birgitta Schmekel. I agree that up to 50 ml appears to sample fluid from the bronchial and larger volumes appears to sample fluid from more peripheral parts of the lung, and as I mentioned this has been visualized by means of digital subtraction radiography. Concerning BAL studies before and after intervention, the alterations of airway wall compliance or bronchodilation by treatment may alter the recovery at least in terms of volumes, but possibly also in term of "protein compartment" sites. I would like to stress, that we need to know more about the kinetics of recovery of fluid phase constituents.

Brattsand. Can we then agree that 50 ml is a suitable volume for BL?

Birgitta Schmekel. I think that by infusing such relatively small volumes into the airways, you lavage the bronchi, and that is one of the very few things that most of us can agree upon concerning lavage technique.

Widdicombe. One possible complication of BL and BAL is that so-called "physiological saline" (0.15 M NaCl) is really a very unphysiological or pathological solution. The liquid lining the airway, when compared to interstitial fluid, is hypertonic, has high potassium and calcium concentrations, and a low pH. 0.15 M NaCl may have powerful actions on the airway epithelium when it replaces the normal airway surface liquid. The changes it induces may influence subsequent lavages. Have you or anyone else compared lavage results with 0.15 M NaCl with those due to more natural lavage liquids?

Birgitta Schmekel. No, I haven't.

Stockley. I have certainly seen data presented at the American Thoracic Society several years ago showing that pH of lavage fluid does affect the results.

Arborelius. When inhaled as an aerosol, both hyper- and hypotonic saline, provoke bronchospasm (and/or coughing) while isotonic saline does not, so in that sense it is physiological also in the airways.

Widdicombe. I agree, but whether or not isotonic saline (0.15 M NaCl) causes physiological effects depends on its site and quantity. It can stimulate reflexes from the larynx and the nose. Perhaps when given as an aerosol it does not cause broncho-constriction because the load and site of deposition are wrong.

Hogg. What can you say about direct comparison between tissue and lavage in animal experiments where tissue changes can be induced with appropriate experimental controls?

Birgitta Schmekel. I'll pass the question to Ralph Brattsand.

Brattsand. Holt, Australia has separated "free" alveolar macrophages from "wall" macrophages and found different properties of them. This is one example that BAL does not sample cells from the "wall parenchyma" or cells firmly adhered to the mucosa.

Persson. I have a comment on the relevance of surface indices to what happens in the underlying airway tissue. Plasma exudation tracers on the mucosal surface seem to reflect extremely well the exudative process in the lamina propria, its intensity and time course.

REFERENCES

Baughman, R.P., Bosken, C.H., Loudon, R.G., Hurtubise, P., and Wesseler, T. (1983) Am. Rev. Respir. Dis. 128, 266-270.

Davis, G.S., Giancola, M.S., Costanza, M.C., and Low, R.B. (1982) Am. Rev. Respir. Dis. 126, 611-616.

Kelly, C.A., Fenwick, J.D., Corris, P.A., Fleetwood, A., Hendrick, D.J., and Walters, E.H. (1988) Am. Rev. Respir. Dis. 138, 81-84.

Kelly, C.A., Kotre, C.J., Ward, C., Hendrick, D.J., and Walters, E.H. (1987) Thorax 42, 624-628.

Lam, S., Lerich, J.C., Kijek, K., and Phillips, D. (1985) Chest 88, 856-859.

Marcy, T.W., Merrill, W.W., Rankin, J.A., and Reynolds, H.Y. (1987) Am. Rev. Respir. Dis. 135, 1276-1280.

Martin, T.R., Raghu, G., Maunder, R.J., and Springmeyer, S.C. (1985) Am. Rev. Respir. Dis. 132, 254-260.

Merrill, W.W., Goodenberger, D., Strober, W., Matthay, R.A., Naegel, G.P., and Reynolds, H.Y. (1980) Am. Rev. Respir. Dis. 122, 156-161.

Merrill, W., O'Hearn, E., Rankin, J., Naegel, G., Matthay, R.A., and Reynolds, H.Y. (1982) Am. Rev. Respir. Dis. 126, 617-620.

Pingleton, S.K., Harrison, G.F., Stechschulte, D.J., Wesselius, L.J., Kerby, G.R., and Ruth, W.E. (1983) Am. Rev. Respir. Dis. 128, 1035-1037.

Rennard, S.I., Basset, G., Lecossier, D., O'Donnell, K., Pinkston, P., Martin, P.G., and Crystal, R.G. (1986) J. Appl. Physiol. 60, 532-538.

Schmekel, B., and Venge, P. Eur. Resp. J., submitted

Schmekel, B., Karlsson, S.E., Linden, M., Tegner, H., Sundström, C., and Venge, P. Inflammation, accepted

11) ASSESSMENT OF SOLUBLE PARAMETERS IN SPUTUM

R.A. Stockley and D. Lomas

Lung Immunobiochemical Research Laboratory, The General Hospital,
Steelhouse Lane, Birmingham B4 6NH, United Kingdom

SUMMARY: The concentrations of soluble protein in lung secretions
are dependent upon the degree of inflammation, local production
and cell activation. Infections and corticosteroid therapy will
alter the protein content of lung secretions as a result of their
effect on lung inflammation.

INTRODUCTION

The sol phase of sputum has been known to contain proteins since
the early studies of Warfringe (1955). These early studies
recognized that many of the proteins were those found in the
plasma. Subsequent workers have identified others such as the
proteinase inhibitor, antileukoprotease (ALP), which is not
present in significant concentrations in plasma. The factors
which affect the amount of these proteins in the lung secretions
will obviously differ depending on their source.

Figure 1 summarizes the possible sources and mechanisms
involved in the passage of proteins into the secretions. Some
proteins such as plasma albumin appear to enter the secretions by
passive diffusion alone. Others, such as the proteinase inhibitor, alpha-1-antichymotrypsin, are made locally by cells within
the lung as well as diffusing from plasma. In some instances

there may be preferential transport mechanisms to facilitate
protein movement into the secretion, such as the secretory
component binding and transport of dimeric Immunoglobulin A. This
latter mechanisms results in a protein that is structurally
different to the plasma derived component. Finally the protein
may be made and released only in the lung and hence will not
present in the plasma.

SOURCE OF BRONCHIAL PROTEINS

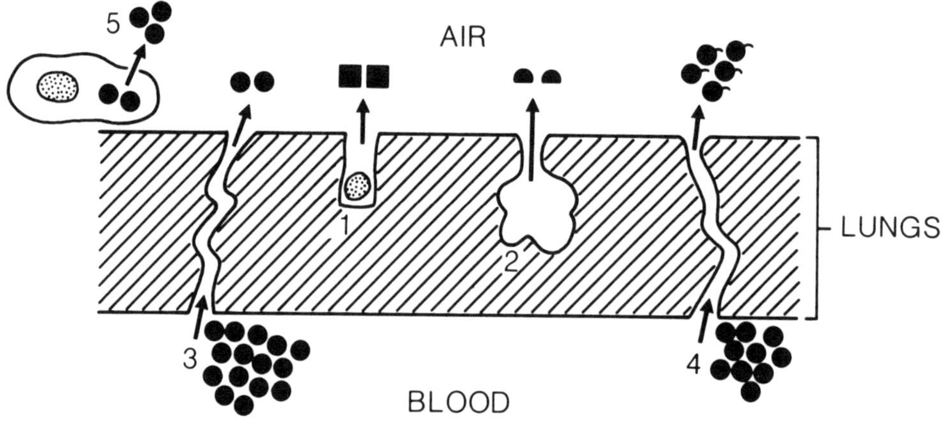

Figure 1. Sources of bronchial proteins: Bronchial
proteins may be derived exclusively from lung cells (1), glands
(2) or by diffusion from plasma (3). In addition active transport
mechanisms (4) and local production by lung cells (5) may enhance
lung concentrations of plasma proteins. (Adapted from Stockley et
al., 1979).

It is critical that the source of the proteins, as well as
factors affecting their behaviour, are taken into account when
assessing the effect of inflammation and monitoring therapeutic
interventions. The plasma derived proteins have been used most

frequently to assess the degree of inflammation as their concentra-tions within secretions are assumed to reflect "leakage" from plasma. However, the choice of protein as well as any "local" contribution from lung cells will affect the results.

FACTORS INFLUENCING SECRETION PROTEINS

Concentration in Plasma: Plasma proteins are largely retained within the vascular space, although a small amount will "leak" through the endothelium into the tissues. The concentration of these proteins in the extravascular space will partly depend upon their plasma concentrations. This is emphasized in Figure 2 for two proteins, albumin and alpha-1-antitrypsin (α-1-AT). The plasma concentrations are approximately 40 and 2 g/l respectively and this is reflected in their sputum concentrations. There is a marked gradient for both proteins and the concentration within sputum are 173.2 (SE ±24.4) and 33.6 (SE ±7.1) mg/l or approximately 0.5-1 % of the plasma concentration. The difference in plasma concentrations is conventionally overcome by use of secretion serum ratios. The results for albumin and α-1-AT are similar as indicated in Figure 3.

Molecular Size: Large plasma proteins will have greater difficulty diffusing into the tissues than smaller proteins unless the degree of lung inflammation is sufficient to allow unrestricted "leakage". This concept has been confirmed for many biological fluids, including the sol phase of sputum (Stockley et al., 1979). The validity of this assumption is confirmed by studies with plasma α-2-macroglobulin (α-2-M) which has a molecular weight of 750,000 daltons. Figure 2 summarizes the plasma and sputum concentrations of this large proteins. The plasma α-2-M concentrations are similar to α-1-AT (1.9 ±0.08 and 2.9 ±0.27 g/l respectively). However, there is almost a 10-fold difference in sputum where the average concentrations in patients with bronchitis are 4.56 mg/l ±1.9 and 33.6 mg/l ±7.1 respectively.

This difference due to size is maintained (although less - see below) even when the plasma secretion ratios are compared as seen in Figure 3 (ratio for α-2-M = 0.3 ± 0.1; ratio for α-1-AT = 1.13 ±0.2).

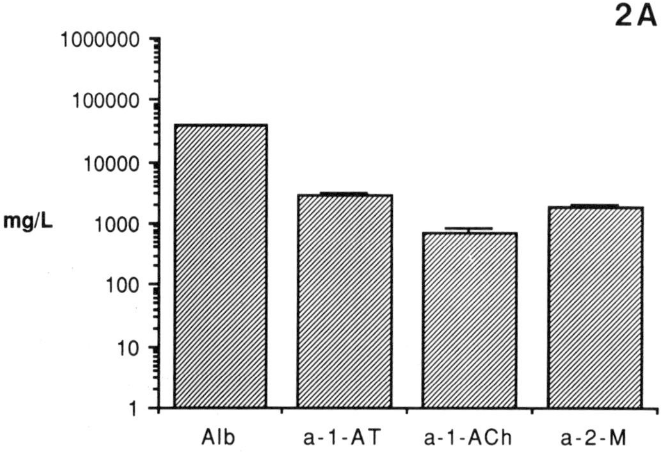

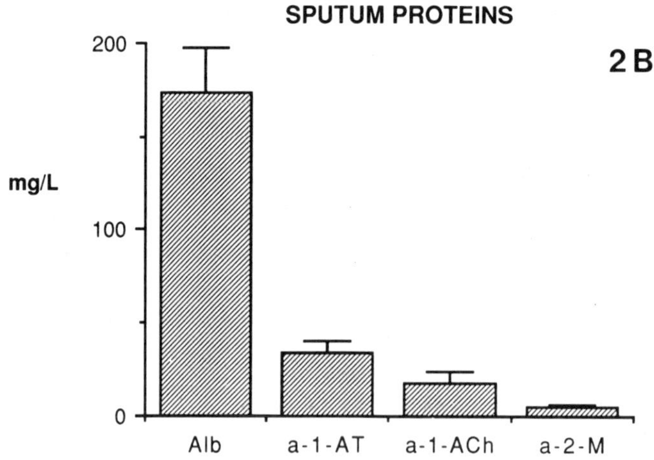

Figure 2. The average serum (2A) and sputum (2B) concentrations are given for the plasma protein albumin (Alb), α-1-antitrypsin (α-1-AT), α-1-antichymotrypsin (α-1-ACh) and α-2-macroglobulin (α-2-M). The bar lines are ± SE.

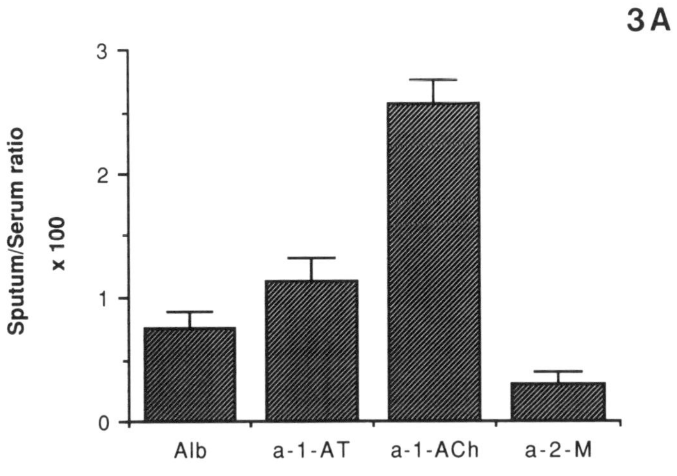

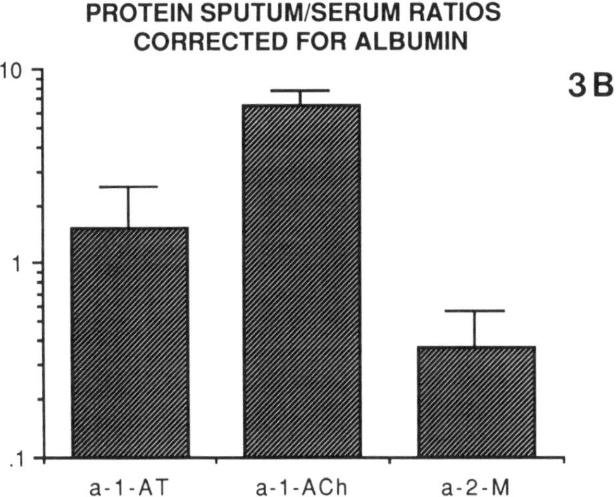

Figure 3. The sputum/serum ratios (± SE) are given (multiplied by 100) for albumin, α-1-antitrypsin, α-1-antichymotrypsin and α-2-macroglobulin (3A). The ratios corrected for (divided by) the albumin ratio are shown in 3B).

Contribution from Local Production: Some plasma proteins including α-1-antichymotrypsin and α-2-M can be produced by alveolar macrophages (Burnett & Stockley, 1984, and White et al., 1981, respectively). Identification of this "local" component is dependent upon finding inappropriately high secretion concentrations for the plasma concentration and degree of protein "leak". In order to determine the protein leak, albumin is taken as the standard on the assumption that no significant quantity is produced in the lung. Thus when the sputum/serum ratio for α-1-ACh is compared to that for albumin a significant difference occurs. This is highlighted in Figure 3, where the average ratio in the absence of infection is 6 times that for albumin. If there was no significant local contribution these ratios would be similar (Stockley et al., 1979).

The situation for α-2-M is a little more complex since the larger size of the protein limits its diffusion into the secretions. However, in view of the relationship between size and diffusion from plasma (Stockley et al., 1979), it has been argued that this protein should be absent from secretions unless it was produced locally in the lung. Thus the presence of α-2-M suggests it is largely the result of local production with a minimal contribution from plasma (Burnett & Stockley, 1981).

Variable Sample Collection: A major problem in the interpretation of protein concentrations in lung secretions has always been variable sample dilution. This may be due to instilled lavage fluid, when obtaining secretions from the lower airways, or saliva and nasopharyngeal secretions when collecting expectorated samples. Many techniques have been utilized to reduce the intra-subject variability due to this dilution.

Correction or standardization for albumin within the sample has been the most commonly used technique. However, although this method does reduce variability for proteins which enter secretions in the same way (by diffusion alone) it is in-appropriate for proteins which are totally or in part produced locally and actually increases variability (Wiggins & Stockley, 1983). Similar problems occur when correcting for total protein content. More recently, standardization for the urea content has been utilized (Rennard et al., 1986) although this may have little advantage over measuring absolute concentrations alone.

These points are emphasized in Figure 4, where the ranking of absolute sputum α-1-ACh concentrations are related to the ranking when corrected for albumin or the urea content. In general, we have concluded that the use of absolute concentrations of sputum/ serum ratios provide the simplest data for the interpretation of changes related to inflammation particularly if the size of the protein and effects of "local" production are taken into account.

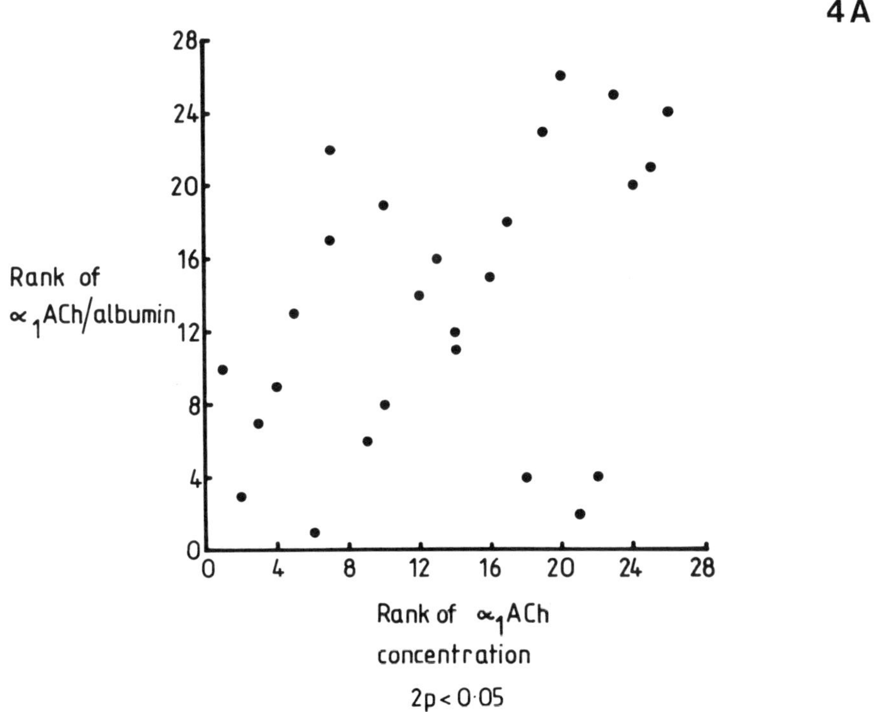

Figure 4A. The ranking of individual sputum sample α-1-ACh concentrations (horizontal axis) is compared to the value corrected for albumin. The significance of the correlation is shown.

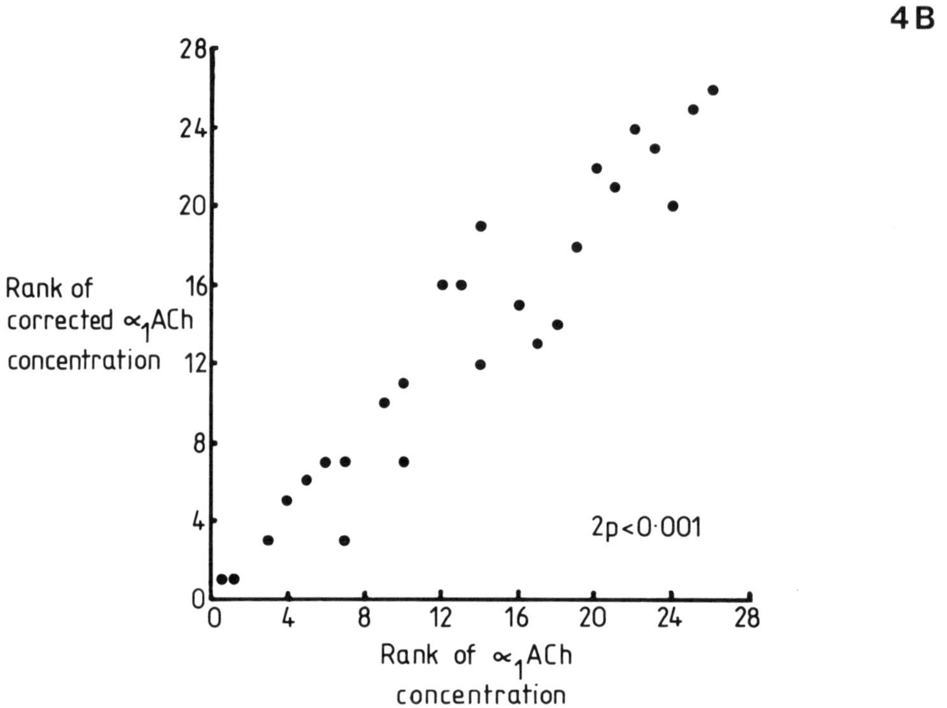

Figure 4B. The ranking of individual sputum sample α-
1-ACh concentrations (horizontal axis) is compared to the value
corrected for the urea content. The significance of the
correlation is shown.

Degree of Inflammation: The presence of inflammation will have
several effects on lung secretion proteins. Some of the plasma
protein concentrations rise as part of the "acute phase"
response. For instance, the concentrations of α-1-AT and α-1-
ACh rise from 2.92 g/l (SE ±0.27) and 675 mg/l (±39.4) to 3.81
±0.36 and 1511 ±125 during infection in patients with chronic
lung disease (Stockley & Burnett, 1979; 1980). This increase
alone will affect the secretion concentrations although the
effect can be overcome, theoretically, by use of the secretion/
serum ratios. However, in addition there is an increased leak
into the lung as indicated by the rise in sputum/serum albumin

ratio seen during infection (from 0.75 ±0.14 to 5.51 ±1.69).

The increase in plasma protein leakage would results in similar changes in the sputum serum ratios of other proteins that are derived predominantly from plasma. For example, the corresponding ratios for α-1-AT rise from 1.13 ±0.20 to 8.22 ±2.61 (Stockley & Burnett, 1979). The similar behaviour for both proteins is confirmed by comparing their ratios. The α-1-AT ratio corrected for (divided by) albumin is 1.52 ±0.1 in the absence of infection and 1.49 ±0.1 during an infection (Stockley & Burnett, 1979).

However, where local lung production provides a substantial contribution towards the secretion concentration during the stable state, different results occur during infection. For instance, although the sputum/serum ratio of α-1-ACh rises during infection from 2.56 ±0.19 to 6.23 ±1.22 comparison with albumin gives very different results. The α-1-ACh ratio "corrected" for albumin actually falls from 6.50 ±1.20 to 2.10 ±0.40 during infection (Stockley & Burnett, 1980). This apparent disparity occurs because the capacity to produce the protein locally is limited. In the absence of infection, there is little protein diffusion from plasma and hence the local component represents a substantial proportion. The sputum/serum ratio is thus inappropriately high for the degree of serum protein "leakage" as reflected in the corresponding albumin ratio. Thus, "correction" for albumin leaves a value much greater than unity.

During infection the lung becomes inflamed and plasma leakage increases as indicated by the rise in sputum/serum albumin. A similar increase in leakage of plasma α-1-ACh occurs, and this plasma derived component swamps the "local" contribution. The α-1-ACh sputum/serum ratio will thus tend to be closer to the ratio for albumin and when divided by the albumin ratio, the result will approach unity.

These processes and results are reversed when the infection settles. During the stable state, there clearly remains a degree of protein "leakage" from plasma. This may reflect a mild degree of inflammation, and this has been confirmed in patients with chronic bronchitis by demonstration of a reduction in the leakage during corticosteroid therapy (Wiggins et al., 1982). Such a reduction in inflammation should be detected by sputum/serum protein ratios that change in the opposite direction to that seen during infection. This is clearly true for sputum proteins that are derived from plasma alone. The albumin ratio falls from 0.46 ±0.06 to 0.34 ±0.06 (results are for last placebo and last treatment day, Wiggins et al., 1982).

A similar change is seen for α-1-AT as reflected in the fact that the sputum/serum ratio falls and when corrected for albumin the result in unaltered (Wiggins et al., 1982). Both proteins are thus behaving in an identical manner. However, again results are different for α-1-ACh because of the "locally" produced component. During steroid therapy the sputum/serum ratio actually rises, and the change is greater when compared to the albumin ratio (Wiggins et al., 1982). These results suggest a significant increase in the "local" contribution with a reduction in the plasma derived component. Indeed, steroids have been shown to increase α1-ACh production by epithelial cell lines (Berman et al., 1988) which reflect one of the sources of the lung protein.

These effects may be easier to monitor for proteins where no significant contribution from plasma occurs. For these proteins comparison with albumin is inappropriate, and absolute concentrations are better to monitor changes during inflammation. For instance, the locally produced inhibitor anti-leukoprotease (ALP) shows a reduction in concentration during infection (when the secretion volume increases) due to a dilutional effect (Dijkman et al., 1986). However, when anti inflammatory agents, such as steroids, are given, the concentration in sputum rises (Stockley et al., 1986a) although it is not known whether this reflects a reduction in the secretion volume, increased local production, or a combination of both mechanisms.

Many other proteins have been studied in secretions including chemotactic factors (Stockley et al., 1988) and Immunoglobulin A (Stockley et al., 1980) which increase in concentration when inflammation is present during infection. In addition, anti-inflammatory agents appear to reduce leakage of carcinoembryonic antigen from the lung into plasma (Stockley et al., 1986b), again indicating a reduction in inflammation.

CONCLUSION: Studies of the soluble proteins in lung secretions can provide useful information on the degree of inflammation. However, it is necessary to be aware that their concentrations and in particular their relationship to each other will depend upon their source and the relative influence of "local" factors within the lung.

DISCUSSION

Widdicombe. A proportion of chronic bronchitics produce no sputum - for example some smokers of low-tar cigarettes. Could you include them in your studies of sputum chemistry by inducing mucus production and expectoration by an appropriate aerosol, such as that of $PGF_{2\alpha}$?

Stockley. I think one could, but I think the technique would need validation. The efficacy and reproducibility will need to be documented. However, I feel that inhalation of prostaglandins or even twice normal saline is likely to effect the secretion constituents. Clearly this could influence the results and direct comparison with sputum would be inappropriate.

Hogg and Hargreave. What is the time course of the sampling of sputum? Is there much variation between single samples and samples pooled over many hours?

Stockley. I'm afraid I cannot provide an answer. We have always collected samples over 4 hours in order to maintain uniformity and obtain a reasonable sample. I think that it is likely that single samples will show more variability than a more prolonged collection.

Venge. We have found that corticosteroids very patently inhibit also the production of chemotactic factors in the lung of asthmatics. Obviously, this parameter is an interesting in vivo reflection of steroid-effects.

Brattsand. Which cells do produce α_1 antichymotrypsin locally?

Stockley. We have shown that alveolar macrophages produce the protein. But it is also present in epithelial cells and we have shown that the T 111 epithelial cell line actively produces the protein. Certainly steroid therapy will increase the α_1 antichymotrypsin production by the T 111 cell line.

Laitinen. What kind of effect does corticosteroids have on the volume of sputum and what was the effect in your studies? How long steroid treatment is required to modulate these sputum soluble parameters?

Stockley. I have no exact data. In the patients I have just described all continued to produce sputum. A reduction in volume would _increase_ the concentrations of sol phase proteins. Despite this possibility the concentrations of albumin fell on steroid treatment suggesting a reduction in inflammations had occurred despite any reduction in sputum volume. The effect of oral steroids occurs within 1 weak. I do not have evidence to confirm whether the effect is maintained or whether it persists after therapy is stopped.

Laitinen. Is the risk increased that CB and COAD patients get pulmonary carcinoma more easily during inhaled corticosteroid treatment?

Stockley. I am not aware that the incidence is increased in asthmatic subjects on corticosteroids. Most lung malignancy is associated with fragile break points on chromosomes. For instance oat cell carcinoma is invariably associated with a deletion on chromosome 3. It is unlikely that steroids would affect this mechanism. However, it is believed that pulmonary macrophages can destroy cells that have escaped from normal differentiation and growth control. Perhaps it is possible that steroids could reduce the efficacy of this surveillance system.

Pride. Do you know of studies of effects of GCS on recurrent infections?

Stockley. Not in smokers/COAD as far as I know.

Brattsand. Are there any close time response studies what is primary and secondary in exacerbations. For instance what appears first in sputum albumin as the marker of inflammation or neutrophils as the marker of infection?

Stockley. I don't think prospective studies have been performed in patients with chronic obstructive bronchitis. This might prove difficult as exacerbations are infrequent. However, previously we did assess patients with cystic fibrosis as out-patients and in-patients with an "exacerbation" (worsening of symptoms). We found no biochemical parameter which predicted the exacerbation or response to treatment. Clearly the patient groups are very different with respect to the severity of the inflammation response.

Larsson. In the Swedish NAC-study, NAC reduced the number of exacerbations. The decline in lung function was, however, not reduced compared to the placebo treated group. This is thus in line with the view that exacerbations have no prognostic importance.

Persson. Judging from the clinical experience with topical airway glucocorticoids, for example in sinusitis, it is the

antiinflammatory action that is most important also in
exacerbations which are believed to be infectious in nature. Old
contraindications for glucocorticoids are thus becoming potential
indications for these drugs.

Gibson. Which is the more crucial factor in exacerbations - the
number of bacteria or the magnitude of the neutrophil infiltrate?
Which should be measured?

Stockley. It is known that the size of the cellular infiltrate
is dependent upon bacterial numbers. Since bacteria are usually
present in the secretion of patients with chronic asthmatic
bronchitis it is likely that an increase in numbers is important.
However, there is no hard evidence available as far as I am
aware. I think that both bacterial number and neutrophil influx
should be measured if possible.

Much of the earlier discussion emphasizes, to me, that the
critical factor is to be sure what we mean by our patient groups
and what an exacerbation of their disease is due to. An
exacerbation means a worsening of something, but this could be
due to superimposed asthma, viral or bacterial infections.
Bacteria are often present in the sputum of patients with chronic
bronchitis even during the stable state. Thus it is difficult to
determine when these bacteria are the cause of an exacerbation.
For steroid intervention we have two possible effects. Either we
can down-regulate an excessive inflammatory response beneficially
as in severely affected cystic fibrosis patients. On the other
hand this is immunosuppressive therapy. Thus it may also increase
susceptibility to infection in some patients.

Bleecker. While there is a tendency to exclude asthma or an
asthmatic tendency one should consider the following: Some
patients may have both an expressive and a host disposition to
asthma as dual etiologies of their airway disease. While these
individuals may be excluded from some studies on chronic airflow
obstruction, patients with these combined etiologies: both asthma

and a chronic decline in FEV_1, associated with cigarette smoking may be a very important group to study.

Jansen. Going back to the problem of defining exacerbations induced by bacterial superinfections I wonder if Dr. Stockley will agree when we will discriminate between infection and colonization in terms of an induced local specific antibody response directed to major antigens epitopes on the microorganism or not. We recently published a study, where we showed a striking local immunoresponse to Haemophilus influenza major epitopes. This was not influenced by short course of corticosteroids, nor that antibiotic treatment had elimination of the persistent microorganism as an effect.

Stockley. Bacteria like Haemophilus express over 20 surface antigens that are detected by the host. We find that local antibody titres are already high in patients with bronchiectasis. A change may occur if a new antigen is expressed by the bacteria or if a different strain enters the lung, but the immune response usually lays behind infection. The IgA system in the lung is, however, a long term response.

Pride. I was surprised to hear you define a significant bronchial infection as one that causes systemic effects. I would think it is possible that damaging airway infections might not be associated with systemic effects.

Persson. There is probably diurnal variations not only in airway secretions but (in airway disease) also in the plasma exudation/ transudation in the airways.

It seems to me that you would like your data to fit with size-selectivity even during acute inflammatory conditions. According to our findings in animal tracheobronchial airways and human nasal airways plasma proteins are exuded in bulk across both the microvascular wall and the epithelial lining. Hence, the inflammatory stimulus-induced plasma exudation/transudation process is largely an unfiltered flow of plasma macromolecules into the airway lumen.

REFERENCES

Berman, G., Burnett, D., Woo, S.L.C., and Stockley, R.A. (1988) Biol. Chem. Hoppe-Seyler, 369 (suppl); 23-26.

Burnett, D., and Stockley, R.A. (1981) Thorax, 36; 512-516.

Burnett, D., and Stockley, R.A. (1984) Am. Rev. Resp. Dis., 129; 473-476.

Dijkman, J.H., Kramps, J.A., and Franken, C. (1986) Chest, 89; 731-736.

Rennard, S.I., Basset, G., Lecossier, D., O'Donnell, K.M., Pinkston, P., Martin P.G., and Crystal, R.G. (1986) J. Appl. Physiol., 60; 532-538.

Stockley, R.A., and Burnett, D. (1979) Am. Rev. Resp. Dis., 120; 1081-1086.

Stockley, R.A., and Burnett, D. (1980) Am. Rev. Resp. Dis., 122; 81-88.

Stockley, R.A., Afford, S.C., and Burnett, D. (1980) Am. Rev. Resp. Dis., 122; 959-964.

Stockley, R.A., Mistry, M., Bradwell, A.R., and Burnett, D. (1979) Thorax, 34; 777-782.

Stockley, R.A., Morrison, H.M., Kramps, J.A., Dijkman, J.H., and Burnett, D. (1986a) Thorax, 41; 442-447.

Stockley, R.A., Shaw, J., Whitfield, A.G.W., Whithead, T.P., Clarke, C.A., and Burnett, D. (1986b) Thorax, 41; 17-24.

Stockley, R.A., Shaw, J., Hill, S.L., and Burnett, D. (1988) Clin. Sci., 74; 645-650.

Warfringe, L.E. (1955) Acta Med. Scand., 153; 49-52.

White, R., Habicht, G.S., Godfrey, H.P., Janoff, A., Barton, E. and Fox, C., (1981) J. Lab. Clin. Med., 97; 718-729.

Wiggins, J., Elliott, J.A., Stevenson, R.D., and Stockley, R.A. (1982) Thorax, 37; 652-656.

Wiggins, J., and Stockley, R.A. (1983) Am. Rev. Resp. Dis., 128; 60-64.

12) SPUTUM CELL COUNTS IN AIRWAY DISEASE: A USEFUL SAMPLING TECHNIQUE

P.G. Gibson, J. Dolovich, J.A. Denburg, A. Girgis-Gabardo, and F.E. Hargreave

Departments of Medicine and Pediatrics, McMaster University and St. Joseph's Hospital, Hamilton, Ontario, Canada

SUMMARY: Quantitative sputum cell counts from patients with asthma and chronic bronchitis were performed and found to be reproducible. Sputum from carefully characterized subjects with asthma contained large numbers of eosinophils and formalin-sensitive metachromatic (mast) cells. In contrast, the macrophage was the dominant cell type in the sputum from smokers with chronic bronchitis. In a third group of patients with corticosteroid responsive-chronic cough and normal methacholine airway responsiveness the sputum contained eosinophils and metachromatic cells, similar to the asthmatic subjects. Sputum cell counts are a useful, noninvasive method for the identification of this pattern of inflammatory response in patients with airway diseases.

INTRODUCTION

The study of airway inflammation promises to deepen our understanding of airway diseases and in particular, airway hyperresponsiveness (Hargreave et al., 1986). The application of indices of airway inflammation to clinical trials is a necessary accompaniment of research into the pathogenesis of airway inflammation. Many of the techniques available for sampling airway inflammatory cells are invasive, requiring bronchoscopy, and this limits their application in clinical trials. Sputum expectoration is a frequent symptom of airway diseases, and the analysis of sputum inflammatory cells may therefore be a useful and noninvasive means of investigating these problems.

Previous studies of sputum inflammatory cells in chronic airflow limitation have given conflicting results. For example, sputum eosinophilia, which is considered a hallmark of allergic asthma, has been reported in smokers with chronic airflow limitation (Vieira & Prolla, 1979; O'Connell et al., 1978) and studies differ as to its association with corticosteroid responsiveness (Shim et al., 1978; Mendella et al., 1982). This has led to the conclusion that sputum analysis was either unreliable or of little utility. These conclusions however are not justified, since in many of these studies the sputum analyses were not quantitative, not demonstrated to be reliable, or there was not careful characterization of the study population. In this article we present the methodology of quantitative sputum cell counts and the results of cell counts obtained from carefully characterized patients with airway diseases.

METHODS

The important features of this method of quantitative sputum analysis, which is a modification of a previously reported technique (Chodosh et al., 1962), are attention to sample collection and particular care applied to selecting a portion of sputum arising from the lower respiratory tract. When attention is given to these aspects, the method can be demonstrated to provide reliable results (Gibson et al., 1979).

Sample collection: Adequate sample collection is essential in order to obtain reliable results. For studies involving comparison between or within subjects, it seems necessary to standardize both the collection time and technique in order to minimize variability in cell counts. This can be done by requesting the collection of early morning sputum samples, promptly transported to the laboratory for processing within 3 hours of collection.

Sample processing: Any sputum sample that is obtained will be a mixture of saliva and lower respiratory tract secretions. In order to obtain information pertaining to the lower airway it is necessary to analyze only those portions of sputum arising from the lower respiratory tract. This can be done by selecting sputum plugs which are shown by microscopy to contain respiratory cells (ciliated epithelium, macrophages) and not squamous epithelial cells. Using an inverted microscope, a sputum plug is chosen with the above characteristics and a total cell count obtained from a portion of the plug suspended in trypsin, stained with crystal violet and then counted in a hemocytometer. A differential cell count may be obtained by directly smearing portions of the same plug onto glass slides and staining with May-Grunwald Giemsa following methanol fixation. Metachromatic cells (mast cells or basophils) may be counted from slides fixed with Carnoy's fluid and stained with 0.5 % toluidine blue at pH 0.5 (Otsuka et al., 1985). Representative counts of eosinophils and metachromatic cells require the evaluation of more than one slide from any one plug and preferably 2 plugs from a sputum sample. The low frequency of metachromatic cells in sputum requires that sufficient cells be counted to obtain an accurate result.

Reliability: In order to evaluate the reliability of quantitative sputum cell counts, we studied subjects (n=15) with chronic cough and sputum who provided early morning sputum samples for analysis on 2 consecutive days (Gibson et al., 1989). Seven subjects were smokers with stable chronic bronchitis and 8 were chronic asthmatic subjects attending the clinic, chosen only by their willingness to submit sputum for analysis.

The results of total and differential cell counts were compared between two plugs selected from the same sample and between 2 samples obtained from the same patient on 2 consecutive days. To prevent observer bias, slides were coded prior to counting so that the investigator was blinded to the clinical characteristics of the subjects. Reproducibility was assessed using analysis of variance with calculation of the reliability coefficient, R, which expresses the variance attributable to within subject differences (error variance) as a ratio of the total variance (Guyatt et al., 1987). R was greater than 0.9 for the total cell count, the eosinophil count and the metachromatic cell count, indicating highly reproducible results (Fig.1). Quantitative sputum cell counts are therefore reliable both between 2 plugs from the same sample, and between 2 samples collected from the same patient on consecutive days.

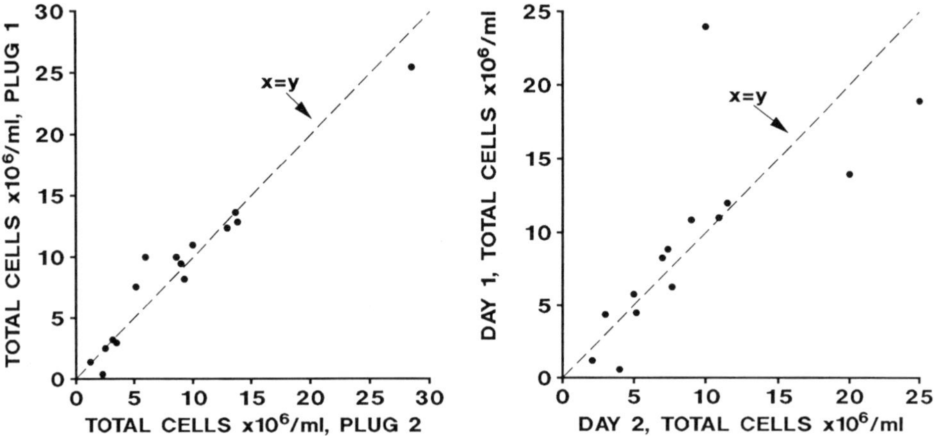

Figure 1: Identity plot of sputum total cell counts showing reproducibility between 2 plugs from the same specimen (left) and 2 specimens obtained from the same patient on consecutive days (right). Sputum cell counts were highly reproducible with reliability coefficients (R) >0.90.

SPUTUM COUNTS IN AIRWAY DISEASES

Asthma and chronic bronchitis: In order to determine the characteristic cellular profile of asthmatic sputum we examined subjects who were carefully documented to have an exacerbation of asthma but no other airway disease (Gibson et al., 1989). They were contrasted with a group of smokers with chronic bronchitis and no clinical features of asthma. Quantitative sputum cell counts were performed, including an analysis of sputum metachromatic cells (mast cells and basophils) which are considered important effector cells in asthma but have not previously been evaluated during an asthma exacerbation. The 10 asthmatic subjects were nonsmokers with methacholine airway hyperresponsiveness (PC20 methacholine < 4 mg/ml) (Hargreave et al., 1986) and an exacerbation of asthma accompanied by sputum (Fig.2, Table I). None was using corticosteroid or cromoglycate in the month prior to study and each had a normal chest x-ray with no evidence of bacterial infection from sputum purulence (grade P3) or antibiotic use in the month prior to or during the study period. Following enrolment and sputum collection the subjects commenced inhaled corticosteroid (beclomethasone 200 μg bid for 2 weeks) and there was complete resolution of sputum and airflow limitation. These subjects were therefore considered to have asthma and no other airway disease. The comparison group comprised 8 smokers with stable chronic cough and sputum. Each had normal spirometry, normal airway responsiveness (PC20 > 8 mg/ml), a normal chest x-ray, and no response to inhaled corticosteroid (beclomethasone 200 μg bid for 2 weeks). They were considered to have chronic bronchitis without evidence of asthma.

The asthmatic sputum was characterized by a marked eosinophilia of (mean ± SE) 69 ± 5 %, and metachromatic cells of 1.5 ± .24 % (Fig.2, Table I). The smokers had significantly less (p<0.05) eosinophils 0.5 ± 0.2 % and metachromatic cells 0.14 ± 0.04 %. The dominant cell in the sputum from smokers was the macrophage which comprised 83 ± 2 % cells. These macrophages had the altered morphologic characteristics previously described in smokers of large multinucleate cells with pigmented cytoplasmic inclusions (Gibson et al., 1989). Sputum total cell counts and differential counts of other cell types were not different between the 2 groups (p>0.05).

Sputum metachromatic cells in the asthmatics were characterized as formalin sensitive mast cells on the basis of light microscopic and histochemical features (Gibson et al., 1989; Otsuka et al., 1985). Basophils were seen in the sputum of only 1 asthmatic subject.

Table I: RESULTS

	Asthma	Corticosteroid Responsive Chronic Cough	Chronic Bronchitis
	n=10	n=7	n=8
Clinical Features			
PC_{20} (mg/ml) mean (range)	0.8 (0.03-3.7)	52.50 (8 - >256)	40.55 (8.6 ->256)
atopy+	8	3	1
smoking	no	no	yes
corticosteroid	yes	yes	no
Sputum Cell Counts			
Total cell count x 106/ml mean (SE)	8.5(2.4)	11.4(2.4)	9.2(1.7)
Eosinophils, %	69(5)	39(10)	*0.5(0.2)
Metachromatic Cells, %	1.5(.2)	1.3(.3)	*0/.14(0.04)

+ number with ≥ 1 positive skin prick to a battery of 12 common
    allergen extracts.
* p < 0.05 vs asthma, chronic cough (ANOVA, Neuman-Keuls).

The results indicate that when subjects are carefully characterized, a distinctive cellular profile is present in asthmatic sputum. Sputum analysis may be useful in the identification of this pattern of inflammatory response in smokers with airflow limitation.

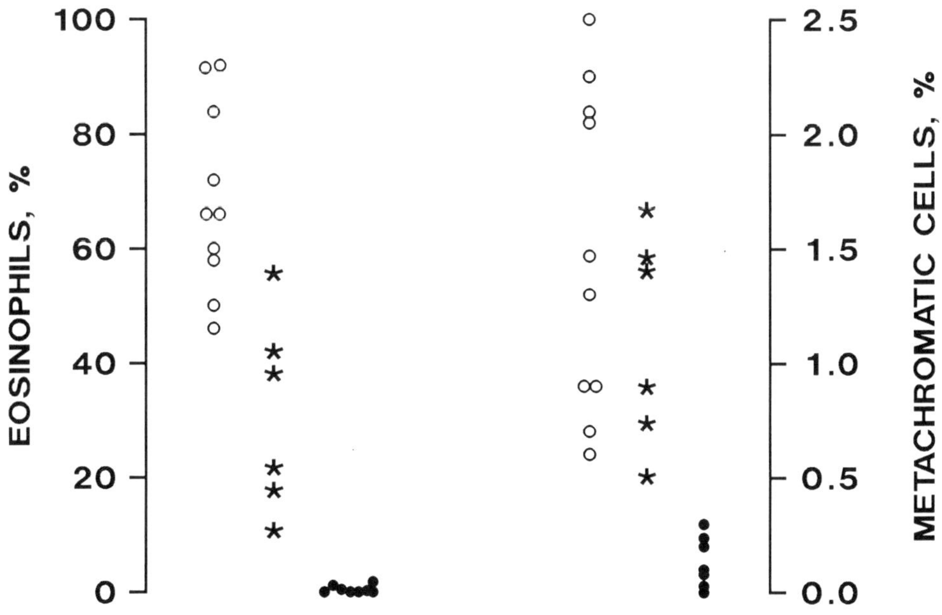

        Figure 2:   Percentages of sputum eosinophils and
metachromatic cells in asthma (O), chronic bronchitis (·), and
non-asthmatic subjects with corticosteroid-responsive cough (*).

<u>Chronic cough</u>: Chronic cough in nonsmokers with normal airway
responsiveness is a not uncommon problem which may respond to
inhaled corticosteroid (Ramsdale et al., 1985). We have examined
sputum from 7 patients with corticosteroid responsive chronic
cough who were identified prospectively from 180 new referrals to
the Firestone Regional Chest and Allergy Clinic (Gibson et al.,
1989). No cause was obvious for the cough.   Each patient had
normal spirometry, normal methacholine airway responsiveness and
a normal chest x-ray. None had evidence of bacterial infection
and post nasal drip was reported by only 2 patients. Sputum was
obtained from these patients prior to corticosteroid therapy and
the cell counts compared with those previously obtained in
chronic bronchitis and asthma (Fig.2, Table I). The corticosteroid responsive chronic cough patients had 39 ± -10 %

eosinophils and 1.3 ± -0.3 % metachromatic cells in their sputum. These values were significantly greater (p<0.05) than observed in the chronic bronchitic patients and comparable to the results of the asthmatic subjects.

The disparity between airway hyperresponsiveness to methacholine and sputum eosinophilia in these patients suggests that infiltration with these cells is, by itself, insufficient for the development of methacholine airway hyperresponsiveness. It may be that cellular activation is also required. Alternatively, the development of sputum eosinophilia may have increased airway responsiveness, but the change occurred within the normal range. This phenomenon has been reported in asthma resulting from occupational exposure to toluene diisocyanate. A further possibility is that the patients are hyperresponsive to other stimuli, such as exercise, but not to methacholine. Further studies are required to examine these possibilities. What shall we call these patients? The available diagnostic terms, asthma and chronic bronchitis, cannot be usefully applied to patients with corticosteroid-responsive chronic cough. They require separate designation from smokers with chronic productive cough, and as they do not exhibit variable airflow limitation, the term asthma cannot be used. This deficiency with current terminology is likely to also be present when examining sputum inflammatory cells in subjects with chronic airflow limitation. Rather than modifying the use of the current terms, it may be useful to describe the salient features with "short hand" labels. Our data suggest that grouping subjects on the basis of common cytological features may be important and the term eosinophilic bronchitis could be used when the eosinophil is the predominant inflammatory cell in the sputum.

APPLICATION TO CLINICAL TRIALS

A stratification variable: Overall these results suggest that the baseline cellular constituents of sputum are likely to have a profound influence on the subsequent response to anti-inflammatory treatment. The presence of sputum eosinophils and metachromatic cells was associated with a favourable response to corticosteroid, irrespective of the presence of airway hyper-responsiveness. Morrow Brown (1958) also reported that sputum eosinophilia was associated with a response to corticosteroid and that the absence of sputum eosinophilia indicated little or no response to corticosteroid . In addition, he suggested that the failure to stratify for sputum eosinophilia was a reason why an MRC trial (1956) unexpectedly found corticosteroid no better than bronchodilator in asthma. Similarly, May (1954) recognized the important confounding effect that sputum eosinophilia could have in clinical trials of antibiotic therapy for chronic bronchitis. He considered sputum cytological examination essential prior to study entry and chose to deal with the problem by excluding such patients from study.

Sputum eosinophilia is a not uncommon finding in chronic bronchitis, being present in up to 30 % of subjects in an unselected series (Miller, 1963). Sputum eosinophilia is therefore likely to be present in a significant number of subjects available for entry into clinical trials of anti-inflammatory therapy in chronic airway diseases. It will influence the response to anti inflammatory treatment, and therefore this variable will need to be identified on entry to such trials and matched evenly between active and placebo treatment groups.

An outcome measure: Many trials of corticosteroid therapy for airway diseases have restricted entry to subjects with chronic airflow limitation and used a measure of airflow limitation as the main outcome assessment (Shim et al., 1978; Mendella et al., 1982). This approach may be inappropriate when the underlying hypothesis considers airway inflammation to be a fundamental abnormality underlying illness. It may be more relevant to consider a measure of airway inflammation as the outcome assessment. One measure of the efficacy of an anti-inflammatory treatment is that it reduces the intensity of the inflammatory cell infiltrate at the site of inflammation. This aspect could be evaluated by sequential evaluation of sputum cell counts. This has been performed in asthma where sputum eosinophils are seen to decrease with corticosteroid therapy of an asthma exacerbation (Baigelman et al., 1983). These results suggest that sputum cell counts may be useful for measuring change over time in clinical trials (Guyatt et al., 1987).

However, prior to their use in clinical trials, further studies are required to document the presence and severity of sputum eosinophilia in smokers with chronic airflow limitation, and to demonstrate the ability of sputum cell counts to detect significant change when it occurs.

Acknowledgements: We thank Mrs. Laurie Whitely for skilful secretarial assistance. The studies were supported by MRC Canada. Dr. Gibson holds a Boehringer Research Fellowship.

DISCUSSION

Laitinen. It is not any more so clear that the sputum is coming only from the bronchial glands. Recently, it has been claimed that a fair amount of sputum is plasma exudation from the bronchial circulation.

Arborelius. Lately, there have appeared a number of papers on "subclinical" asthma, characterized by night cough and dyspnea but with normal FEV_1 and no increase in FEV_1 after $ß_2$-agonists. However, they respond to $ß_2$-stimulants and inhaled corticosteroids. They probably have bronchospasm confined to small airways. In 10 normal subjects Volume of Trapped Gas (VTG) increased by 100 % without any change in FEV on 1 mg methacholine/ml. In 20 subjects with isocyanate exposition VTG increases from 100 ml to 550 ml on the same provocation with a mean decrease in FEV_1 of only 5 %.

Gibson. In future studies, it will be important to examine the small airways in more detail. The observations remain, however, that in the chronic cough patient we were unable to demonstrate variable airflow limitation. They therefore cannot be described with the term asthma.

Persson. Could it be that your patients having glucocorticoid-sensitive cough but no sign of asthma were subjects that soon will develop manifest asthma? I am asking this because cough may be the first sign in children who develop asthma.

Gibson. Yes, it is possible.

Löfdahl. You showed data from Brown, 1958, demonstrating that the effect of corticosteroids is dependent on eosinophilia, and you argued that sputum eosinophilia is an important parameter to use in stratification in a long-term interaction study with a corticosteroid. I think that those data could be applied to short-term studies, preferentially in asthma patients. I doubt whether this is applicable in a long-term study of e.g. the corticosteroid effect on COAD, which we discussed yesterday. In such a study I think we study another pathogenetic mechanism than in asthma.

Do you really think sputum eosinophilia has to be used for stratification in such a study?

Gibson. The presence of sputum eosinophilia is associated with a favorable response to glucocorticoid. Because this variable has bearing on subsequent treatment response, it must be considered and handled appropriately, for example by balancing subjects with sputum eosinophilia between active & placebo treatment groups.

Koeter. Was the cough in your patients induced by allergen exposure or by viral infections?

Gibson. All the patients had chronic cough and sputum for greated than 3 months. This is longer than what would be expected for an acute viral infection. Three patients were atopic, one of them had a history of seasonal exacerbations in symptoms.

Persson. Your comparison between asthmatics and bronchitics is very interesting but you may have to study both groups under similar conditions. So my question is: do you know of sputum characteristics and steroid effects on cough in your bronchitics under exacerbations?

Gibson. No.

REFERENCES

Baigelman, W., Chodosh, S., Pizzuto, D., and Cupples, L.A. (1983) Am. J. Med. 75, 929-936.
Brown, H.M. (1958) Lancet ii, 1245-1247.
Chodosh, S., Zaccheo, C.W., and Segal, M.S. (1962) Am. Rev. Respir. Dis. 85(5), 635-648.
Gibson, P.G., Girgis-Gabardo, A., Morris, M.M., Mattoli, S., Kay, J.M., Dolovich, J., Denburg, J., and Hargreave, F.E. (1989) Thorax Vol 44, No. 9, 693-699.
Gibson, P.G., Dolovich, J., Denburg, J., Ramsdale, E.H., and Hargreave, F.E. (1989) Lancet i, 1346-1348.
Guyatt, G., Walter, S., and Norman, G. (1987) J. Chron. Dis. 40(2), 171-178.
Hargreave, F.E., Dolovich, J., O'Byrne, P.M., Ramsdale, E.H., and Daniel, E.E. (1986) J. Allergy Clin. Immunol. 78, 825-832.
May, J.R. (1954) Lancet ii, 839-842.
Medical Research Council. (1956) Lancet ii, 798-803.
Mendella, L.A., Manfreda, J., Warren, C.P.W., and Anthonisen, N.R. (1982) Ann. Intern. Med. 96, 17-21.
Miller, D.L. (1963) Am. Rev. Respir. Dis. 88, 473-483.
O'Connell, J.M., Baird, L.I., and Campbell, A.H. (1978) Respiration 35, 65-72.
Otsuka, H., Denburg, J., Dolovich, J., Hitch, D., Lapp, P., Rajan, R.S., Bienenstock, J., and Befus, D. (1985) J. Allergy Clin. Immunol. 76(5), 695-702.
Ramsdale, E.H., Morris, M.M., Roberts, R.S., and Hargreave, F.E. (1985) In: Glucocorticosteroids, Inflammation and Bronchial Hyperreactivity (J.C. Hogg, R. Ellul-Micallef and R. Brattsand, Eds), Excerpta Medica, Amsterdam, pp. 91-96.
Shim, C., Stover, D.E., and Williams, M.H., Jr. (1978) J. Allergy Clin. Immunol. 62(6), 363-367.
Vieira, V.G., and Prolla, J.C. (1979) J. Clin. Pathol. 32, 1054-1057.

13) BRONCHIAL BIOPSIES IN DRUG INTERVENTION STUDIES IN CB AND COAD

Annika Laitinen[1], L. A. Laitinen[2], and T. Haahtela[3]

[1]Department of Medical and Physiological Chemistry, University of Lund, Sweden and Department of Electronmicroscopy, University of Helsinki,Finland, [2]AB Draco, Explorative Clinical Research, Lund, Sweden, [3]Department of Allergic Diseases, Helsinki University Central Hospital, Finland

SUMMARY: So far, little information is available on the usefulness of the biopsy method in drug intervention studies in COAD and CB. Quantitation studies at electron microscopical level are time consuming. Comparative studies between and within the patient groups are needed to attain basic and clinically relevant information. Pathology studies may lead to a better understanding of basic pathophysiological mechanisms behind the diseases.The sequence of cellular events could be revealed so that morphology may be useful in intervention studies.

INTRODUCTION

Since there is a lack of information of airway pathology, chronic obstructive airway diseases (COAD) have been diagnosed based on clinical observations and physiological respiratory function measurements. The limitations of these methods have led to diagnostic confusion in the group of COAD: asthma, chronic bronchitis and emphysema. Very little has been known of the pathological changes in these diseases as well as the basic mechanisms involved in each disease (Laitinen, 1989, Reid et al., 1989, Laitinen & Laitinen 1990a, 1990b).

A classically important tool, histology, has not been used much because of the difficulties in obtaining specimens in living patients and because of lack of motivation. The possibility of pathological changes in the airways in COAD at an early stage of the disease has been denied. The developments in the bronchoscopic and ultrastructural electron microscopic techniques have been essential to attain knowledge of airway morphology in COAD.

Taking bronchial biopsy specimens is one possible method used to study the efficacy of anti-inflammatory drugs in COAD. In order to get valuable information, the bronchial biopsy specimens should be taken, processed and analyzed by a standardized method. (Laitinen & Laitinen, 1988).

METHODOLOGICAL DIFFICULTIES ASSOCIATED WITH BRONCHIAL BIOPSY STUDIES

Difficulties in obtaining specimens: Obtaining representative specimens from the human airways underlies the main problem of morphological studies. Bronchitic or asthmatic patients seldom have lung surgery. Thus, biopsies form the only possibility to study fresh airway specimens. So far, we have very little information of the usefulness of ultrastructural morphological studies of asthmatic or bronchitic airways in relation to clinical practice (Laitinen, 1985; Laitinen et al., 1985; Lundgren et al., 1988; Beasley et al., 1989; Jeffery et al., 1989).

Lung surgery in chronic bronchitis and emphysema is due to pulmonary infiltrates seen in x-ray pictures or identified lung cancer usually in a late phase of the disease (Wright et al., 1988). There is no knowledge of possible early morphological changes at ultrastructural level in either patient group.

Presently, there is practically no experience of the usefulness of histology and electronmicroscopy as a possible tool in helping to diagnose COAD. Only a few studies to examine airway morphology using bronchial biopsies have been conducted in patients with chronic obstructive pulmonary disease (Glynn & Michaels, 1960; Dunnill et al., 1969; Cutz et al., 1978; Laitinen et al., 1985; Lundgren et al., 1988; Beasley et al., 1989; Jeffery et al., 1989). These morphological studies have revealed early changes, especially in asthma, recognizable at ultrastructural level.

Co-operation between the clinic and the histology unit: Since obtaining comparable material is obscured by the diversity of the disease itself, as well as the treatment used, careful patient characterization is essential for all biopsy studies. Direct contacts between the clinician and the morphologist are valuable in avoiding methodological problems in the handling of the specimens. Procedures causing artefactual destruction of the biopsies can be diminished by proper biopsy technique, immediate fixation and careful handling of the specimen. The choice of fixative is important because of the small size of the specimen. It may be difficult to divide the specimen for different fixatives.

Table I. Technical problems related to receiving fresh biopsy specimens by bronchoscopy

- should the patient be hospitalized or not?

- local anaesthesia versus general anaesthesia

- fiberoptic versus rigid tube bronchoscopy

- definition of the airway levels studied

- complications of the bronchoscopy procedure

Light microscopy versus electron microscopy: Using light microscopy, larger areas of the biopsy or surgical specimens can be studied. However, because of the limitations in the magnification with this method, little information of the fine structure of the individual cells (e.g. epithelial cells, vascular endothelial cells) and structures usually not visible by small magnifications, such as nerves, can be achieved.

Another difficulty lies in recognizing different kinds of inflammatory and other mobile cells. Their recognition in light microscopy is usually based on their different staining properties. In disease states, however, these cells can also show changes in morphology such as degranulation, which is difficult to evaluate without studies at the ultrastructural level (Laitinen, 1989).

In electron microscopy, the magnitude of the specimen is much more restricted than in light microscopy. Since the specimen is introduced into the microscope on a special grid in a holder, the size of the grid is a limiting factor for all EM quantitation. Conventional grids contain small copper bars, which help to support the specimen on the grid, and no other special cover is needed. This leads the grid to be a network usually with 100 to 300 small openings. The size of one opening is limited to approximately 50x50 to 200x200 square micrometers depending on the mesh number. The grid bars being approximately 30 micrometers thick, highly limit the view under electronmicroscopy. This is especially disturbing when one tries to study all the 300 openings, as the human epithelium in the specimen is, to some extent, curved. Even about 60 % of the specimen may be hidden behind the grid bars.

A special cover has to be developed if the grid opening is to be used as one big whole. The cover must be thin enough not to disturb the contrast in the pictures, and tolerable enough so that the thin section lying on it will not be broken. If a strong enough cover can be developed, the whole area of the grid can be used, and the thin section can be studied and photographed as a whole under electron microscopy.

The use of the conventional grids usually means that a total number of cells with more or less limited identification has to be studied in the much larger histological section. These numbers are then extrapolated to electronmicroscopy, for example, by counting the "first hundred " recognized cells in the different holes in the EM section (Beasley et al., 1989). However, if comparisons are made between groups of patients, such as controls and a diseased group, this quantitation may lead to misinterpretation of the results. If the density of the total number of cells is smaller in the control group than in the diseased group, larger areas have then to be studied under electron microscopy to achieve the first hundred identified cells. If the correlation between the total number of cells counted in light microscopy is made to the proportion of individual cells achieved in counting the first hundred cells, this may lead to a higher proportional finding of one particular cell in the controls only because a larger area has to be used to find the first hundred cells.

In order to avoid confusion between different morphological studies, the methods used should be stated in a precise way, and if possible the quality, as well as the size of individual specimens, should be visualized in the study produced by the quantitative electron microscopy. Otherwise, the readers do not know the basis from which all the information for statistical analysis is achieved.

When using larger uniform areas of airway mucosa containing several hundreds of epithelial cells in the section, several problems still arise. Even a one millimeter long area in the airways is extremely small. How does the limited finding correlate to the universal situation in the airways? More studies correlating findings from two or more airway levels are needed.

Despite how small the specimen is in comparison to the whole airways, it represents the changes (due to the real disease) at the moment the biopsy was taken . This can be useful in trying to find and develop animal models to study COAD. It may also lead to recognition of cells and their interactions. By studying successive biopsies, patient groups with different duration of the disease may give more information of the sequence of cellular events in the tissue.

OWN RESULTS WITH BRONCHIAL BIOPSY STUDIES

Our recent studies from bronchial biopsies from living asthmatics show that different kinds of epithelial changes may occur in asthmatic airways: close to normal epithelium with inflammatory cells, goblet cell hyperplasia with or without ciliated cells, metaplasia and shedding of the epithelium. Goblet cell hyperplasia which can also occur in chronic bronchitis may reflect a common nonspecific reaction of the epithelium to an irritant. The difference in the irritant to the epithelium may lead to further differences in the course of the disease in COAD, because shedding of the airway epithelium and infiltration with mast cells and eosinophils are rare in smokers. In early stages of asthma, an inflammatory process to unknown stimulus causes an infiltration of a mixture of cells to the epithelium (mast cells, eosinophils and lymphocytes) and the lamina propria (eosinophils, lymphocytes, plasma cells and macrophages) when compared to control subjects. Also the airway microcirculation shows changes in asthmatics compared to controls. Asthmatics show endothelial disruptions, gaps in the venular endothelium, and leucocytes in the blood vessels, probably reflecting chemotaxis of these cells.

Morphological studies have revealed early changes in asthma recognizable at ultrastructural level. The developing inflammatory process at the early stage of the disease involves mainly eosinophil, lymphocyte and plasma cell infiltration of the lamina propria, and especially mast cells in the epithelium. Neutrophils do not occur during the early development of the disease. Neutrophils were observed in higher numbers only in severe asthmatics with several years of clinical disease and may thus reflect a more complicated disease. The morphological studies have given insight to COAD with respect to both treatment and animal models.

CONCLUSION: We conclude that with increasing experience of quantitative morphological studies we may in the future, be able to determine the effects of drugs on the cellular picture of the airways.

DISCUSSION

Hogg.   First of all I would like to compliment you on a very elegant study. Do you observe any differences between COAD and asthma in terms of where the increased wall thickness occurs? I wonder whether it might be submucosal in asthma and evenly distributed throughout the wall in COAD?

Annika Laitinen. With bronchoscopy we do not get specimens deep enough to permit a comparable measurement of the thickness of the airway wall.

Chung.   Could you tell us, in your experience, the differences you find between biopsies obtained by the rigid bronchoscope and those from the fibre optic bronchoscope, as most people use the latter technique?

Annika Laitinen.   When we have studied biopsies taken with a fibre optic bronchoscope, it has been difficult to get representative specimens from the airway epithelium. By fibre optic bronchoscopy the tissue beneath the epithelium - the lamina propria - can be studied.

Venge.   We have very recently completed a study on asthmatic patients, together with Jean Bousquet in France. In this study a large number of patients were lavaged and biopsied. It is very clear from this study that the number of eosinophils in the lavage and the tissue is greatly increased and correlated to the severity of the disease. This is obviously at variance with your findings. Do you think that you have difficulties identifying the eosinophils in your sections?

Annika Laitinen.   The numbers of eosinophils shown today only apply to the airway epithelium. As part of a larger study, we have been able to study biopsies from the same asthma patients at a stable stage and during the acute phase of the disease. In the stable stage, no eosinophils were detected in the epithelium. In the biopsies taken during the acute phase, the epithelium and lamina propria were filled with eosinophils, also showing morphologically features of degranulation, such as loss of the crystalloid core protein in the granules. This gives some evidence that the presence or absence of eosinophils in the airways may reflect a dynamic process related to disease activity.

Hargreave. Eosinophils in BAL are often not raised in stable mild asthma, while there are small increases in mast cells. Where, exactly, was the site of the bronchial biopsies?

Annika Laitinen. Biopsy 1) From the right upper lobe bronchus Biopsy 2) From the opening of right middle or lower lobe Biopsy 3) From the subsegmental carina of a first order segmental bronchus.

REFERENCES

Beasley, R., Roche, W.R., Roberts, J.A., and Holgate, S.T. (1989) Am. Rev. Respir. Dis. 139, 806-817.
Cutz, E., Levison, H., and Cooper, D.M. (1978) Histopathology 2, 407-421.
Dunnill, M.S., Massarella, G.R., and Anderson, J.A. (1969) Thorax 24, 176-179.
Glynn, A.A. and Michaels, L. (1960) Thorax 15, 142-153.
Jeffery, P.K., Wardlaw, A.J., Nelson, F.C., Collins, J.V., and Kay, A.B. (1989) Am. Rev. Respir. Dis. 140, 1745-1753.
Laitinen, A. (1985) Thorax 40, 488-492.
Laitinen, L.A., Heino, M., Laitinen, A., Kava, T., and Haahtela, T. (1985) Am. Rev. Respir. Dis. 131, 599-606.
Laitinen, L.A., Laitinen, A. (1988) Eur. Respir. J. Vol. 1, No. 5, 488-489.
Laitinen, L.A., Laitinen, A. (1990a) In: Pharmacology of Asthma, Handbook of Experimental Pharmacology. (C. P. Page and P.J. Barnes, Eds.) Springer Verlag (in press).
Laitinen, L.A., Laitinen, A. (1990b) In: The Lung, Scientific

Foundations. (R.G. Crystal, J.B. West, P.J. Barnes, and E.R. Weibel Eds.). Raven Press (in press).

Laitinen, L.A. (1989) In: Glucocorticoids and Mechanism of Asthma. (I.E. Hargreave, J.C. Hogg, J.L. Malo, amd J.H. Toogood. Eds.) Excerpta Medica, pp 215-229.

Lundgren, R., Söderberg, M., Hörstedt, P., and Stenling, R. (1988) Eur. Respir. J. 1, 883-889.

Reid, L.M., Gleich G.J., Hogg, J., Kleinerman, J., and Laitinen, L.A. (1989) In: The role of inflammatory processes in airway hyperresponsiveness. (S. Holgate, Ed.) Blackwell Scientific Publications, pp 36-79.

Wright, J.L., Hobson, J.E., Wiggs, B., Pare, P.D. and Hogg, J.C. (1988) Lung 166, 277-286.

14) INFLAMMATORY INDICES FOR CHRONIC BRONCHITIS AND CHRONIC OBSTRUCTIVE AIRWAY DISEASE. CELL POPULATIONS IN BRONCHIAL AND BRONCHOALVEOLAR LAVAGE.

Margareta Linden[1], J.B. Rasmussen[2,3], Eeva Piitulainen[3], M. Larsson[4], and R. Brattsand[1].

[1]Laboratory of Pharmacology, Research & Development Department, AB Draco, Box 34, S-221 00 Lund, Sweden, [2]University of Lund, Institution of Pulmonary Medicine, Malmö, Sweden, [3]Department of Pulmonary Medicine, Malmö General Hospital, Malmö, Sweden, [4]Medical Department, AB Draco, Lund, Sweden.

SUMMARY: The development of chronic bronchitis (CB) and chronic obstructive airway disease (COAD) seems to be related to inflammatory changes of airway structure. However, the cause and the exact location and type of these changes resulting in altered airway function are not known. Mucosal inflammation is characterized by the recruitment of granulocytes, macrophages and lymphocytes as well as by the shedding of epithelial cells. The present chapter discusses the usefulness of bronchial lavage (BL; 50 ml of lavage volume) directly followed by bronchoalveolar lavage (BAL; 200 ml), for the characterization and quantification of inflammation in proximal and peripheral airways, respectively. On the basis of results from the literature and a pilot study on CB patients with or without coexisting COAD, the following conclusions may be drawn:
 - There is a profound difference in lavage cell composition and numbers between non-smokers and smokers. However, within the group of smokers there are few additional changes in cell numbers and composition when concomitant airway disease is present.
 - The obstruction of the COAD patients is correlated to a reduced recovery of BL and BAL fluid. Furthermore, these patients seem to have a reduced number of most cell types in their BL. This diminitution is not just related to the reduced fluid recovery.

- The BL cells have a lower viability and BL macrophages have
a reduced phagocytic capacity when compared with matching BAL
cells. The viability of cells was lowest in BL from the COAD
group. These findings may suggest that COAD entails a reduced
transport of macrophages to the small airways and/or an enhanced
turnover of these cells in the bronchi.
- Functional studies of lavage cells may supply additional,
and perhaps more specific, information on the mechanisms involved
in the inflammatory process.

INTRODUCTION

Chronic bronchitis (CB) is a clinical syndrome defined as the
production of excessive secretions by the tracheobronchial tree.
There is a strong association between cigarette smoking and the
development of CB and irreversible airways obstruction. Functional and morphological investigations of small and large
airways in CB suggest that airway inflammation is the earliest
abnormality found in smokers, and that this inflammation may
contribute to the development of CB and of the sometimes
concomitant chronic obstructive airway disease (COAD) (Reynolds
& Merrill, 1981; Mullen et al., 1985).

Bronchoalveolar lavage (BAL) is an important research instrument in various diseases affecting the lung (Crystal et al.,
1986; Reynolds, 1987). This technique makes it possible to
investigate types and numbers of inflammatory cells recruited
into the airway lumen, e.g. in bronchitic patients. Such studies
may be useful in elucidating the mechanisms of airway diseases,
and they may be useful in monitoring disease activity in longitudinal studies, as well. The presence of airway inflammation in
CB is supported by studies which demonstrate markedly enhanced
numbers of total cells, alveolar macrophages and sometimes
neutrophils in BAL obtained from cigarette smokers (Davis et al.,
1982; Hunninghake & Crystal, 1983). However, there is very little
in the way of comparable lavage data from patients with CB, with
and without airways obstruction. To our knowledge, the only published study was performed by Martin et al. (1985). However, the
group of obstructive patients included in this study was hetero-

geneous, which makes proper comparisons difficult. Properly
designed lavage studies comparing CB patients with and without
obstruction may be useful in elucidating the probably partly
dissimilar inflammatory processes underlying CB and COAD.

LOCATION AND TYPE OF AIRWAY INFLAMMATION IN CB AND COAD

By determining the clinical status and pulmonary function in
bronchitic patients before they underwent lung operations, it has
been possible to some extent to relate the respiratory problems
to the type and localization of airway inflammation. With regard
to bronchitic patients who still have FEV_1 and FVC within the
normal range, the study by Mullen et al. (1985) described inflammatory changes in the mucosa, submucosa and glands of the airways, particularly the cartilaginous ones with a luminal diameter
of ≥ 3 mm, while slighter changes were seen in smaller airways. It
is reasonable to conclude that the secretion, cough and exacerbation symptoms of CB are related to the enhanced vascular exudation, glandular secretion and metaplasia of ciliated epithelium
within this airway region.

Approximately 20 % of the patients fulfilling the clinical
criteria of CB will develop an irreversible obstruction. In the
present discussion, the combined occurrence of CB symptoms and
irreversible airways obstruction is referred to as chronic
obstructive airways disease (COAD). Even though inflammation also
seems to contribute to the obstruction, clinical as well as
histopathological evidence suggests that the problems associated
with secretion-cough and obstruction are actually different
processes with regard to the type and the site of inflammation.
Clinically, there is no close correlation between the extent of
secretion-cough and the prospective development of obstruction;
in fact, a high secretion rate is often a good prognostic sign in
the active treatment of COAD (Peto et al., 1983; Anthonisen et
al., 1986). Functional studies have shown that the main site of
increased airways resistance in COAD-patients is the small

conducting airways, especially the respiratory bronchioles (Cosio et al., 1978). Morphologically, such airways demonstrate an increased number of inflammatory cells (mainly macrophages), increased connective tissue deposition in the airway wall, epithelial metaplasia and decreased support from adjacent alveoli (Cosio et al., 1978; Mullen et al., 1985; Wright et al., 1988; Hogg 1990 - this volume). All these inflammatory changes will contribute to the enhanced airflow resistance of COAD, and a recent study has shown that these types of inflammation persist even after cessation of smoking (Wright et al., 1988).

THE LIMITATIONS OF LAVAGE AS A SAMPLING METHOD
FOR AIRWAY INFLAMMATION

Earlier studies using BAL demonstrate the presence of inflammation in the airway lumen of bronchitics, with a large influx of macrophages and also some recruitment of neutrophils (Reynolds & Merrill, 1981; Mullen et al., 1985). One obvious limitation on the part of the lavage technique per se, is that only the free luminal cells and the easily-detached epithelial cells can be sampled. Furthermore, the conventional BAL performed with a total volume of 200-250 ml has a low sampling selectivity, where the airways are concerned, because the majority of cells collected originates from the vast alveolar surfaces.

The value of lavage sampling would be much greater if more selective sampling could be performed within the central cartilaginous airways, the small airways and the alveoli, respectively. This would make for a better identification and quantification of various inflammatory processes underlying the secretion-cough, the obstructive and the emphysema symptoms. More selective airway sampling can, in fact, be achieved by a single washing with 50 ml (Lam et al., 1985; Schmekel, 1990 - this volume). The airway deposition of this volume is verified by digital substraction radiography (Kelly et al., 1987) and by the altered differential cell count (higher proportions of neutrophils and epithelial cells; Lam et al., 1985; Schmekel, 1990 - this volume). However, in practice, some inevitable mixing of airway and alveolar con-tents could occur. The specificity of sampling just the large-airways content may be further increased by using 5-20 ml as a lavage volume (Lam et al., 1985). However, the recovery of such small lavage volumes is too low for cell functional studies.

The aim of this chapter is to discuss the possibility of obtaining more specific information about the airway inflammation in CB and COAD by means of combining bronchial lavage (50 ml) and consecutive bronchoalveolar lavage (200 ml). The discussion is based on results from a pilot study in CB patients with or without coexisting obstruction (COAD).

PATIENT SELECTION AND SAMPLING OF BRONCHIAL (BL) AND BRONCHO-ALVEOLAR LAVAGE (BAL)

Sixteen patients, fulfilling the clinical criteria of CB (Medical Research Council, 1965), were recruited and divided into two groups depending on their level of airway obstruction. The patients (n=9) without appreciable obstruction had FEV_1 >75 % of predicted value (96 ±6 %; mean ±SEM), and the bronchitics with coexisting obstruction (n=7) had FEV_1 <75 % of predicted value (51 ±6 %). All were current smokers (26.7 ±3.0 and 32.6 ±10.6 pack-years, respectively). The mean age was 53 ±4 years in the non-obstructive and 47 ±3 years in the obstructive group.

The lavage was performed similarly to the one described earlier by Linden et al. (1988), i.e. by means of instilling five 50-ml aliquots of sterile saline into the main bronchus of the middle lobe. However, the first-aspired aliquot (BL) was processed separately from the four following ones, which were pooled in one container (BAL). The recovery of BL and BAL fluids was recorded. After the centrifugation of lavage fluids, the cells were resuspended and the cell viability (Trypan blue exclusion), the total (Burker chamber) and the differential cell counts (cytocentrifuge preparations stained with May-Grunwald Giemsa) were estimated in a manner that has been described previously (Linden et al., 1988). The differential cell counts (1000 cells/ sample) included alveolar macrophages, neutrophils, eosinophils, basophilic cells, lymphocytes and epithelial cells. Because of differences in the lavage fluid recovery between the CB and COAD groups (Table I), the numbers of various cell types are presented both as the total number (Table I) and as the concentration (Table II).

The functional status of the macrophages was determined by their ability to phagocytose fluorescein-labelled yeast particles (Linden et al., 1988). The phagocytic capacity of macrophages obtained from BL was compared to that of the ones obtained from BAL. In most BLs from obstructive bronchitics, however, the number of macrophages was too low for this test.

Table I. Recovery of lavage fluid and cells in patients with chronic bronchitis. Data represent the mean ±SEM. BL = bronchial lavage; BAL = bronchoalveolar lavage.

		NON-OBSTRUCTIVE (n=9)		OBSTRUCTIVE (n=7)	
		BL	BAL	BL	BAL
FLUID RECOVERY	(%)	34±3	68±2°°°	20±5*	44±6***°
CELL VIABILITY	(%)	65±7	91±1°°	40±14	77±7
TOTAL CELL NUMBER ($\times 10^6$)		17.7± 14.4	71.1±° 10.5	1.8± 0.7	45.6± 20.5
MACROPHAGES	(%)	84.0± 2.7	94.8± 0.9	60.1± 14.4	93.5± 1.8
($\times 10^6$)		15.3± 12.4	67.8± 10.4	1.1±* 0.4	44.0± 20.2
NEUTROPHILS	(%)	7.2± 2.0	2.1±° 0.4	5.9± 2.2	2.0± 0.6
($\times 10^6$)		1.03± 0.87	1.30± 0.24	0.10± 0.04	0.76± 0.36

contd/

		NON-OBSTRUCTIVE (n=9)		OBSTRUCTIVE (n=7)	
		BL	BAL	BL	BAL
EOSINOPHILS	(%)	2.89± 1.46	0.60± 0.27	2.02± 0.98	0.25± 0.06
$(x10^6)$		0.38± 0.26	0.39± 0.16	0.02± 0.01	0.10± 0.05
BASOPHILIC CELLS	(%)	0.15± 0.08	0.08± 0.05	0.19± 0.19	0.07± 0.04
$(x10^6)$		0.04± 0.04	0.05± 0.03	0.01± 0.01	0.01± 0.01
LYMPHOCYTES	(%)	1.36± 0.49	1.93± 0.63	0.52±* 0.20	2.87±°° 1.00
$(x10^6)$		0.16± 0.11	1.23±°° 0.38	0.01± 0.01	0.68± 0.26
EPITHELIAL CELLS ciliated	(%)	2.54± 0.68	0.23±° 0.09	11.10± 9.16	1.38± 0.74
$(x10^6)$		0.56± 0.49	0.17± 0.05	0.45± 0.42	0.14± 0.05
squamous	(%)	1.91± 0.72	0.31± 0.21	3.48± 0.99	0°
$(x10^6)$		0.23± 0.18	0.21± 0.17	0.06± 0.02	0°

* p<0.05; ** p<0.01; *** p<0.001 non-obstructive bronchitics and obstructive bronchitics compared using Mann-Whitney U test for unpaired data.
° p<0.05; °° p<0.01, °°° p<0.001 BL and BAL compared using Wilcoxon's signed rank test for paired observations

CELL POPULATIONS IN LAVAGE

BAL in non-obstructive bronchitics: Rough comparisons with earlier BAL studies can be made here. However, no parallels are drawn to previous results described for "healthy smokers", as it is - in our opinion - difficult to make a clear distinction between this group and bronchitics.

The BAL fluid recovery (68 %) and the cell viability (91 %) in BAL from the bronchitics (Table I) are comparable to those of healthy non-smokers (Linden et al., 1988). Thus, there is no valid support for the assumption that the large airways of these patients are obstructed with regard to fluid, and that their luminal cells possess decreased viability, when they are lavaged during an exacerbation-free period. However, the total cell count in BAL (71×10^6) is much higher than in healthy non-smokers (16×10^6; Linden et al., 1988), indicating the presence of inflammation in the bronchitic airways.

The differential cell count is similar to previously reported findings in smokers (Davis et al., 1982; Hunninghake et al., 1983), with a predominance of alveolar macrophages (95 %), while the proportions of neutrophils (2 %), lymphocytes (2 %) and epithelial cells (0.5 %) are all low (Table I). In healthy non-smokers, the corresponding proportions are 87 %, 1 %, 10 % and 2 %, respectively (Linden et al., 1988). Thus, although the proportions of cells are rather similar in these two clinically different groups, the absolute counts are several times higher in the bronchitics.

<u>Bronchial Lavage (BL) in non-obstructive bronchitics</u>: This lavage (50 ml) yielded a fluid recovery of 34 %. Even though this figure is only half that of BAL (p<0.001; Table I), it is comparable to the recovery of BL in healthy non-smokers (40 %, Schmekel, 1990 - this volume). This shows that the low fluid recovery in the BL of bronchitics is an effect caused more by anatomical-technical factors than by pathophysiological changes.

There was a significant difference between BL and BAL in respect of the viability of the recovered cells (Table I). While the viability of the BAL cells was 91 %, it was only 65 % (p<0.001) for the cells recovered in BL (Table I). This difference does not apply only to bronchitics. In healthy non-smokers too, the cell viability in BL is mere 69 % (Schmekel & Linden, in preparation). However, a clear distinction between bronchitics and healthy non-smokers is valid regarding the total number of cells in BL: 18×10^6 and 2×10^6 cells were recovered in bronchitic (Table I), and non-smoking subjects, respectively (Schmekel & Linden, in preparation). Although the cell proportions are quite similar in these two groups, with about 85 % macrophages, 7-11 % neutrophils and 2-5 % epithelial cells, the bronchitic airway mucosa was thus covered with about 10 times more cells.

BAL in obstructive bronchitics: Fluid recovery was much lower ($p<0.001$) in the obstructive (44 %) than in the non-obstructive patients (68 %; Table I), showing that the obstruction not only refers to air but also to the passage of fluid. The viability (77 %) and the total cell count (46×10^6) of the obstructive group tended to be lower than the values for the non-obstructive patients (90 % and 67×10^6, respectively). The proportions and absolute counts of macrophages, neutrophils, eosinophils, basophils and lymphocytes, were approximately the same in the two groups (Tables I and II). In the obstructive group, however, squamous epithelial cells were totally absent (Tables I and II).

BL in obstructive bronchitics: Even in this compartment, the mean of fluid recovery (20 %) was significantly lower than in the non-obstructive group (34 %; $p<0.05$). Cell viability (40 %) in the obstructive group also tended to be lower than that in the non-obstructive bronchitics (65 %; Table I). Ten times fewer cells (1.8×10^6) were collected by the BL of the obstructive subjects (Table I), and in fact, this number is comparable to the number of cells collected by BL from healthy non-smokers (2×10^6, Schmekel & Linden, in preparation). Due to the very large variation within the non-obstructive group, there was no significant difference with respect to the total number of cells between the non-obstructive and obstructive groups. However, the number of alveolar macrophages was significantly lower in the BL of the obstructive group ($p<0.05$; Table I).

Table II: Cell concentrations in lavage obtained from patients with chronic bronchitis. Data represent the mean ±SEM. BL = bronchial lavage; BAL = bronchoalveolar lavage.

	NON-OBSTRUCTIVE (n=9)		OBSTRUCTIVE (n=7)	
	BL	BAL	BL	BAL
TOTAL CELLS $(x10^4/ml)$	85.0± 65.0	57.0± 8.0	16.0± 6.0	44.0± 16.0
MACROPHAGES $(x10^4/ml)$	72.8± 56.2	53.9± 8.0	9.8± 2.4	42.0±° 16.2
NEUTROPHILS $(x10^4/ml)$	4.98± 3.90	0.98± 0.14	0.78± 0.24	0.77± 0.29
EOSINOPHILS $(x10^4/ml)$	1.98± 1.23	0.43± 0.25	0.19± 0.09	0.10± 0.04
BASOPHILIC CELLS $(x10^4/ml)$	0.21± 0.17	0.06± 0.04	0.08± 0.08	0.01± 0.01
LYMPHOCYTES $(x10^4/ml)$	0.84± 0.49	1.05± 0.36	0.13± 0.10	0.82± 0.31
EPITHELIAL CELLS ciliated $(x10^4/ml)$	2.63± 2.22	0.16± 0.07	4.47± 4.17	0.27± 0.13
squamous $(x10^4/ml)$	1.12± 0.81	0.17± 0.14	0.57± 0.22	0 °

° $p<0.05$; BL and BAL compared using Wilcoxon signed rank test for paired observations.

This large difference in the number of BL macrophages - much greater than one would have anticipated as a result of the somewhat lower fluid recovery in the obstructive group - is surprising and needs to be confirmed in a larger group of patients. As was stated above, there was no significant difference in BAL-macrophage counts between the two groups. This difference with respect to the bronchial cell number is unexpected, as both groups had bronchitic problems and the common hypothesis (see Introduction) is that these problems are related to the extent of bronchial inflammation. However, it is proposed that the low number of bronchial macrophages in BL obtained from the obstructive individuals may reflect the obstruction of the small airways. The majority of bronchial macrophages is recruited from the peripheral airway compartments. The inflammatory process underlying the peripheral obstruction may inhibit the transport of macrophages from the alveoli to the bronchial region in at least two ways. The obstruction may cause some physical hindrance or, perhaps more importantly, the AMs may become more activated and adhesive at the inflammatory site and therefore, become "trapped" in small airways. A higher extent of activation is supported by the finding that the secretion of pro-inflammatory mediators (e.g. PGE_2 and IL-1β) in cultures of AMs obtained from the obstructive bronchitics was higher than that of AM cultures from the non-obstructive patients (Linden et al., 1990).

PHAGOCYTIC CAPACITY OF ALVEOLAR MACROPHAGES FROM BL AND BAL

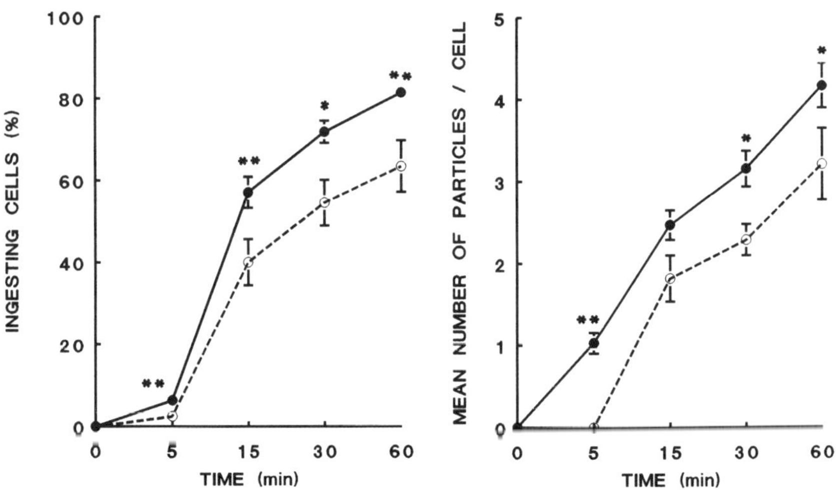

Figure 1. Alveolar macrophages obtained by BL and BAL from patients with chronic bronchitis (n=9) were purified by adherence to a glass surface. The phagocytic capacity of adherent macrophages was studied by means of the ingestion of fluorescein-labelled yeast particles (Linden et al., 1988). The results are expressed as mean ±SEM. A statistical comparison between macrophages from BL (-⊖-) and macrophages from BAL (-●-) was performed, using Wilcoxon's signed rank test for paired observations. *: p<0.05; **: p<0.01.

Besides this reduction in the absolute macrophage count from the obstructive group, there were tendencies to reduced absolute numbers, by a factor of 5-10; this applied to the granulocytes and lymphocytes, too (Table I). Calculated as differential counts, the lymphocyte proportion was lower (p<0.05), whereas the percentage of squamous epithelial cells tended to be higher.

COMPARISON OF FUNCTIONAL ACTIVITY OF MACROPHAGES IN BL AND BAL

The phagocytosis activity (Fig. 1) and the cell viability (Table I) indicate a significantly impaired activity on the part of the BL compared to the BAL macrophages. This suggests that the macrophages of the bronchi represent a deteriorating population cleared from the alveoli, or that the "mucoid" environment of the bronchi may bring about an impairment of AM function.

CONCLUSION: The composition of bronchial and bronchoalveolar lavages demonstrate an ongoing airway inflammation in smoking bronchitics (Reynolds & Merrill, 1981; Martin et al., 1985, Terpstra et al., 1987, present study). The inflammation is verified by the presence of 5-10 times more cells, especially macrophages, neutrophils, lymphocytes and epithelial cells (the latter indicating enhanced epithelial turnover), in bronchitic patients than in healthy non-smoking individuals. However, these changes seem to be rather non-specific, as "healthy smokers", bronchitics and bronchitics with coexisting airway obstruction have a similar cellular profile (Reynolds & Merrill, 1981; Martin et al., 1985, Terpstra et al., 1987, Linden et al., 1988).

In the pilot study reported here, we have investigated whether combined bronchial and bronchoalveolar lavage may be a more sensitive method for the monitoring of inflammation in the bronchial and peripheral compartments, respectively, of the airways. The study needs to be extended to include larger patient groups. However, the preliminary results indicate that the coexisting presence of airway obstruction in CB patients is accompanied by discrete changes in the cell counts. The most remarkable finding was a lowered number of AMs in the bronchi of the COAD patients.

Additional information can be supplied by functional studies of the lavage cells, e.g. AMs. Such studies suggest that the obstruction may be related to an increased pro-inflammatory activity on the part of these cells (Linden et al., 1990).

DISCUSSION

Gibson. Which measurement contains the greatest variance, or spread of data, bronchial washings or bronchoalveolar lavage ? If BAL data is tighter, would it not be a better sampling technique ?

Margareta Linden. The greatest variance is obtained with bronchial lavage because of mucus which may cause heterogenous cell distribution within the sample.

The answer to your second question is yes. However, the important point is that different compartments are monitored by lavaging with the small and large lavage volumes, respectively.

Birgitta Schmekel. Concerning the spread of data in bronchial lavage, this may also depend on the variability in smoking habits and the resulting variability of inflammatory response.

Stockley. I was very interested in your data on lavage neutrophils. The percentage differential count in BAL was lower than in BL. However, the absolute numbers were the same. This suggests that neutrophils are a feature of BAL but the data can be hidden by the increased return of macrophages in BAL thus reducing the percentage of neutrophils.

Laitinen. How would you and Birgitta Schmekel value the usefulness of BAL or BL in intervention studies?

Margareta Linden. Rather few differences in cell counts were observed in this study. BAL may be more useful as a source of inflammatory cells for functional studies.

Birgitta Schmekel. The clinical relevance of BL and BAL and the diagnostic power of the method to predict clinical course in terms of therapeutic effects have caused considerable controversy. There are obvious limitations of the method and reproducability may be a bit of a problem. However, there are ways to overcome, at least partly, the problem by for example lavage in several bronchi using exogenous and/or endogenous markers etc. But we do need to know more about kinetics of the recovery of soluble substances (and we should try to correlate the BAL-result to other more conventional lung function parameters).

REFERENCES

Anthonisen, N.R., Wright, E.C., and Hodgkin, J.E. (1986) Am. Rev. Respir. Dis. <u>133</u>, 14-20.

Cosio, M., Ghezzo, H., Hogg, J.C.,Corbin, R., Loveland, M., Dosman, J., and Macklem, P.T. (1978) N. Engl. J. Med. <u>298</u>, 1277-1281.

Crystal, R.G., Reynolds, H.Y., and Kalica, A.R. (1986) Chest <u>90</u>, 122-131.

Davis, G.S., Giancola, N.S., and Constanza, M.C. (1982) Am. Rev. Respir. Dis. <u>126</u>, 611-616.

Hunninghake, G.W., and Crystal, R.G. (1983) Am. Rev. Respir. Dis. <u>128</u>, 833-838.

Kelly, C.A., Kotre, C.J., Ward, C., Hendrick, D.J., and Walters, E.H. (1987) Thorax <u>42</u>, 624-628.

Lam, S., Leriche, J.C., Kijek, K., and Phillips, D. (1985) Chest <u>88</u>, 856-859.

Linden, M., Wieslander, E., Eklund, A., Larsson, K., and Brattsand, R. (1988) Eur. Respir. J. <u>1</u>, 645-650.

Linden, M., Rasmussen, B., Larsson, M., Piitulainen, E., Brattsand, R., and Laitinen, L.A. (1990) Am. Rev. Respir. Dis. <u>141:4</u>, A646.

Martin, T.R., Raghu, G., Maunder, R.J., and Springmeyer, S.C. (1985) Am. Rev. Respir. Dis. <u>132</u>, 254-260.

Medical Research Council Committee on the Aethiology of Chronic Bronchitis (1965) Lancet <u>i</u>, 775-779.

Mullen, J.B.M., Wright, J.L., Wiggs, J.L., Pare, P.D., and Hogg, J.C. (1985) Br. Med. J. <u>291</u>, 1235-1239.

Peto, R., Speizer, F.E., Cochrane, A.L. Moore, F., Fletcher,

C.M., Tinker, C.M., Higgins, I.T.T., Gray, R.G., Richards, S.M., Gilliland, J., and Norman-Smith, B (1983) Am. Rev. Respir. Dis. 128, 491-500.

Reynolds, H.Y. (1987) Am. Rev. Respir. Dis. 135, 250-263.

Reynolds, H.Y., and Merrill, W.W. (1981) Med. Clin. N. Am. 65, 667-689.

Terpstra, G.K., Wassink, G.A. and Huidekoper, H.J. (1987) Int. J. Clin. Pharm. Res. VII, 357-361.

Wright, J.L., Hobson, J.E., Wiggs, B., Pare, P.D., and Hogg, J.C. (1988) Lung 166, 277-286.

15) THE GENERATION OF REACTIVE OXYGEN-DERIVED SPECIES BY PHAGOCYTES

H. Bergstrand

The Pharmacological Laboratory, AB Draco, Box 34, S-221 00 Lund, Sweden.

SUMMARY: The generation of reactive oxygen-derived species is one main constituent of the microbicidal activity of professional phagocytes. This process is known as the respiratory or the oxidative burst. It is initiated by a cyanide- and azide-insensitive increase in O_2-consumption and the concomitant generation of superoxide radicals catalyzed by a membrane-localized NADPH oxidase which is triggered by an appropriate stimulation of the cells. The generated O_2^- is converted to hydrogen peroxide, hydroxyl radicals and other reactive products of oxygen which, if released extracellularly (for example in connection with frustrated phagocytosis), are potentially harmful to the tissue. The oxidative burst is not necessarily dependent on phagocytosis, nor is it necessarily associated with degranulation. Therefore, the process constitutes an important independent variable of phagocyte activity, and researches aiming to characterize various forms of airway inflammation may derive valuable information from an examination of the oxidative burst.

INTRODUCTION

When appropriately triggered professional phagocytes - i.e. monocytes, macrophages, neutrophils and eosinophils - respond by a marked increase in oxygen consumption. This respiratory or oxidative burst (OB) is not inhibited by blockers of the mitochondrial respiration, such as cyanide or azide. It is due to the activation of a plasma membrane-localized, normally dormant, oxidase which catalyzes the one-electron reduction of oxygen to superoxide radicals at the expense of NADPH generated in the hexose monophosphate shunt (cf Fig.1). The superoxide radicals are converted mainly in phagocytic vacuoles into hydrogen peroxide, hydroxyl radicals and other reactive products of oxygen, such as hypohalites and chloramines. These products are part of the phagocytes' armour for microbicidal purposes. If inappropriately released from the cell (e.g. in connection with frustrated phagocytosis), they are potentially harmful to the tissue of the host. The primary effects of these oxygen-derived agents include the purported oxidation of proteins, making them autoantigenic and/or highly susceptible to proteolytic attack.

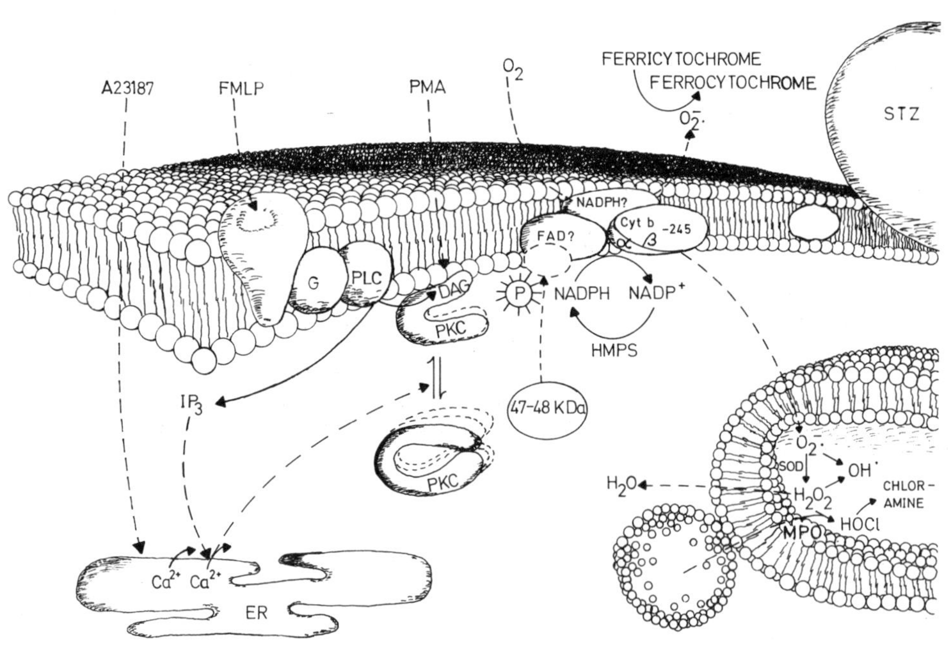

Figure 1. Schematical representation of the concepts of the phagocyte oxidative burst.

The oxidative burst is not necessarily dependent on phagocytic events, nor does it have to be associated with degranulation. It seems to be a unique process which may be triggered and modulated independently of other phagocyte functions.

The purpose of the present paper is to supply a brief overview of the OB. The discussion concerning the molecular basis of this process chiefly refers to findings regarding neutrophils; studies on the OB activity of bronchoalveolar (BAL) phagocytes mainly reflect that of macrophages. For details and appropriate literature citations, the reader is referred to recent comprehensive reviews (Babior, 1987; 1988; Bellavite, 1988; Borregaard,1988; Rossi, 1986; Segal, 1989).

ASSAY

The oxidative burst can be measured in vitro as oxygen consumption (with the aid of an oxygen electrode); as superoxide-mediated ferricytochrome-C reduction (change in absorbency at 550 nm); as H_2O_2-mediated oxidation and concomitant loss of fluorescence of scopoletin, catalyzed by horse-radish peroxidase; and as the generation of hydroxyl radicals, detected by any one of the following means: the degradation of deoxyribose; as the chemiluminescence enhanced by lucigenin (superoxide dependent) or by luminol (hydrogen peroxide and myeloperoxidase dependent); or as the intracellular reduction of nitroblue tetrazolium (NBT). It is more difficult to demonstrate generation of oxygen-derived reactive species in vivo; the most often used principle in this respect is electron paramagnetic resonance measurements and spin trapping.

The NADPH oxidase: The enzyme system responsible for the oxidative burst is the NADPH oxidase. The characterization of this oxidase is presently the focus of very intensive research among several groups. This is a hard task because the enzyme is highly instable.

The NADPH oxidase is found only in professional phagocytes. A severe disorder, chronic granulomatous disease (CGD) - characterized by serious predisposition to protracted bacterial infections - is associated with a lack of phagocyte NADPH oxidase activity due to defects in one or more of the putative components of the enzyme.

The evidence today favors participation in the oxidase-catalyzed reaction of the following components: a cytochrome, a flavoprotein, a NADPH-binding component and a cytosolic 47-48 KDa protein. Whether these components are all separate, is a matter of some dispute. The oxidase is normally dormant in the cell. In activated cells, however, it is chiefly localized in the cell membrane. The location of the different components of the inactivated enzyme has not been unequivocally determined.

The cytochrome has a low redox potential, - 245 mV, and an α-band of light absorption at 558 nm. It is, therefore, referred to as cytochrome b_{-245} or cytochrome b_{558}. It has been purified and shown to be composed of the heme and two protein subunits, an α chain of 23 kDa and a glycosylated ß chain whose molecular weight is 76-93 kDa. The genes for both these chains have been cloned; the sequences show little resemblance to other mammalian cytochromes. Interestingly, the α-subunit is apparently transcribed but not translated in non-phagocytes. The reason for this is not clear. Both chains of the cytochrome b_{-245} seem to be phosphorylated during superoxide generation; these phosphorylations are kinetic-ally not associated with activation of the NADPH oxidase, but they might be involved in cessation of the activity.

A flavoprotein with a FAD prosthetic group is also probably a component of the oxidase. Whether this protein is identical to a 66-67 kDa putative NADPH-binding protein of the oxidase is a matter of controversy; another not mutually exclusive possibility is that the flavoprotein is identical with a 47-48 kDa cytosolic protein, phosphorylated at an early point in the process of activation of the oxidative burst. However, recent results question the membrane localization of the NADPH-binding component of the oxidase in inactivated cells. The 66-67 KDa membrane-associated protein may not be the oxidase-associated NADPH-binding subunit (Smith et al., 1989). The 47-48 KDa cytosolic protein is partially translocated to the cell membrane after phosphorylation; this translocation is apparently a "docking" of it to the cytochrome b_{-245}. The protein after this translocation seems to undergo further phosphorylations. Recent experiments with antibodies against the activated oxidase identify a 16/18 kDa and 14 kDa heterodimer, whose function has not been clarified (Berton et al., 1989).

CGD patients of the X chromosome-linked category lack both chains of the cytochrome; the defect has been pinpointed as occurring in the gene coding for the ß chain. Patients of the autosomal recessive category seem to express both chains normally; however in these patients the 47-48 KDa protein is not appropriately phosphorylated. Either it may be missing, or the pertinent serine or threonine residue(s) may be displaced by mutation.

Activation of the oxidative burst: Activation of the NADPH oxidase in vitro can be accomplished by triggering cells using various particulate stimuli, such as serum-treated zymosan (STZ) or soluble, receptor-associating stimuli like FMLP, LTB_4, C5a and PAF. More artificial ones, such as phorbol ester (e.g. PMA) or a calcium ionophore (e.g. A23187) are often utilized to trigger the burst in vitro. The utilized signal-transduction pathways seem to vary along with the different stimuli that have been employed and the different cells that were examined. However, at least in the neutrophil, the signal initiated by most secretagogues possibly ends up in the stimulation of protein-kinase-C (PKC) activity and the phosphorylation of the 47-48 kDa cytosolic component. FMLP and fluoride (presumably acting through G protein[s]) can evidently trigger neutrophil oxidative responses which are not clearly dependent on an increase in the intracellular levels of calcium and/or diacylglycerol and PKC activation (Rossi et al., 1989).

Protein-kinase-C is heterogenous; at least seven isozymes are now described which are encoded by different genes and are differentially expressed in different cells. These isozymes of PKC are apparently differentially modulated by the second messengers diacylglycerols and calcium (Nishizuka, 1988). Which PKC isozyme that would be responsible for the phosphorylation of the cytosolic 47-48 kDa component is not clear. Available reports suggest that the main PKC form of neutrophils is similar to either the α- or the β- isozyme. Minor PKC forms can also be observed in neutrophils (Olsson & Bergstrand, 1989).

The issue of whether superoxide radical generation is electro-genic, leading to a cytoplasmic accumulation of protons which, if not pumped out of the cell, will lead to an inactivation of the burst, is controversial (Naccache et al., 1989).

Activation of the NADPH oxidase in subcellular systems: Activation of the NADPH oxidase can also be accomplished in suitably reconstituted subcellular systems by means of arachidonic acid or detergents like SDS. In this system, PKC activity does not seem to be a necessary link in the signal-transduction pathway, as phorbol esters express low activating efficacy and activation can be accomplished in the virtual absence of ATP. Activation in the subcellular system calls for a membrane component and possibly four or even five different cytosolic components (Curnutte et al., 1989).

Priming of cells for an oxidative burst: When challenged, neutro-phils in suspension respond with a transient burst of radical generation, whereas adherent cells respond according to a much more protracted time course. This implies major differences in the control of the burst in these situations (Nathan 1987; 1989). The phagocyte has to be suitably primed to be able to respond at appropriate triggering with an optimal oxidative burst. With regard to human macrophages, gamma-interferon has been reported to be a necessary and sufficient primer; other cytokines such as GM-CSF and TNF as well as somatotropin have also had priming properties attributed to them (Bass et al., 1989; Edwards et al., 1989; Koenderman et al., 1989). Gamma-interferon treatment and TNF treatment of CGD neutrophils synergistically lead to increased mRNA transcript levels of cytochrome b_{-245}. The neutrophil is reportedly primed by LPS for enhanced oxygen-radical generation by LPS as well, but recent findings suggest that LPS could also block the PMN respiratory burst.

The mechanism(s) for the priming of the OB are not clarified; but phosphorylation and/or fatty acylation of components of the oxidase, followed by their translocation to the plasma membrane, are possible events in this process. Granulocytes primed with GM-CSF respond with a respiratory burst to increases in the cytosolic level of calcium; in cells harvested from blood, such an event is not in itself sufficient to trigger the cells (Sullivan et al., 1989)

Pharmacological modulation of the oxidative burst: An inhibition of the oxidative burst in vitro can be seen in the presence of specified putative protein-kinase-C inhibitors such as staurosporine, in the presence of certain amphiphilic drugs like the naphthalene sulfonamide W-7 and in the presence of the putative intracellular calcium antagonist TMB-8. Ketotifen and azelastine are drugs which reduce phagocyte radical generation in vitro. These agents presumably act at the level of the secretagogue signal transduction. Diphenyl iodonium blocks the activity of the FAD-binding protein of the NADPH oxidase; it is a more potent inhibitor of this oxidase than of the mitochondrial correspondent.

Compounds inhibiting or counteracting the priming of phagocytes would also be interesting pharmacological tools for the modulation of NADPH oxidase activity. We are not aware of any agents with this activity except the following ones: (i) endotoxin/LPS, which impairs the monocyte formation of reactive oxygen metabolites (Rellstab & Schaffner, 1989) and, in trace levels, prevents interferon-gamma or TNF-alpha to enhance macrophage respiratory-burst capacity (Ding & Nathan 1987); (ii) tumor-cell-conditioned medium; and (iii) beta-interferon, which reportedly counteracts the effect of gamma-interferon and alpha-interferon which reduce the transcription rate of the NADPH oxidase ß-chain.

On the other hand, it is noteworthy that several reports fail to record substantial inhibition of the OB as a result of GCS-treatment, both in vitro and in vivo. It is also noteworthy that inhalation of ozone (1 ppm for 3 hr) leads to a decreased capacity of mouse alveolar macrophages to produce superoxide radicals (Ryer-Powder et al., 1988). This is not seen in humans at 0.4 ppm ozone for 2 hr (Koren et al., 1989).

Tissue injury induced by the oxidative burst: The degree to which reactive oxygen species are involved in various pathological conditions is not clarified (cf Weiss, 1989). One reason for this is the lack at the clinical level of drugs that specifically reduce this process (to our knowledge, no drug is unequivocally shown to act in humans by reducing the oxidative burst). However, the observation that phorbol esters, highly potent and effective stimuli of the process, are extremely effective inflammation-inducing agents in animals in vivo suggest an important role for the oxidative burst in inducing tissue damage at the site of inflammation. The role of oxygen-derived reactive species may even be a primary one; an oxidant attack on proteins may transform them into auto-antigens and/or increase their susceptibility to degradation by proteolytic agents.

Oxidative response of BAL phagocytes: BAL-cell oxidative responses can be assessed either directly after a harvest of cells with the aim of catching an ongoing process, or after some form of culture geared to enriching adherent cells. The possible influence on cellular response of the local anaesthesia employed when performing BAL has to be considered in the former procedure; in the latter, the possible in-vitro restoration of any aberrant activity must be taken into account. In both approaches, it is desirable to utilize several secretagogues thought to act through different signal-transduction pathways such as STZ, immune complexes, C5a, FMLP and even artificial ones such as a phorbol ester and a calcium ionophore. The influence of subject age should be compensated for; in rabbits, the O_2^--generating capacity of neonatal alveolar macrophages is substantially lower than that of cells from adult animals (Sherman & Lehrer, 1984)

Below I will summarize some reported aspects on BAL phagocyte oxidative burst and airway-disease activity.

Table I. BAL phagocyte oxidative activity and airway disease.

Condition	Finding
Smoking	BAL phagocytes show increased OB at stimulation
Silicosis Asbestosis	Increased spontaneous and stimulated BAL cell OB response
Sarcoidosis	- " -
Interstitial lung disease	- " -
RA	- " -
Asthma	Increased stimulated BAL phagocyte OB
Chronic Air-flow disease	Correlation between degree of bronchial hyperreactivity (histamine) and peripheral blood PMN superoxide generation (PMA)

It is now generally agreed that BAL cells from smokers show increased radical generation, regardless of the conditions under which this process is followed (adherent cells or cells in suspension) (Bergstrand et al., 1986; Richter et al., 1986; Marcy & Merrill, 1987). This increased radical generation by smokers alveolar macrophages inactivates the α1-antitrypsin activity in epithelial lining fluid; it could thus play a role in the pathogenesis of emphysema associated with smoking (Hubbard et al., 1987).

Inhalation by humans or experimental animals of organic dusts (for example asbestos, quartz or cotton-bract extract) may lead to a priming of lung inflammatory cells for PMA-triggered O_2^--generation (Cantin et al., 1988; Cooper et al., 1988). The chronic inflammatory response of asbestosis and silicosis are characterized by increased spontaneous alveolar-macrophage superoxide and hydrogen-peroxide generation (Rom et al., 1987).

Alveolar macrophages from sarcoid patients examined in suspension culture immediately after bronchoalveolar lavage or after adherence purification, release increased amounts of H_2O_2 or superoxide spontaneously or after challenge with PMA (Fels et al., 1987; Calhoun et al., 1988).

BAL cells from children as well as adult patients with interstitial lung disease (ILD) show increased spontaneous and PMA-triggered superoxide or H_2O_2-production compared with cells from normal individuals (Cantin et al., 1987; Clement et al., 1987). It is suggested that oxidants together with myeloper-oxidase play a part in causing the epithelial-cell injury associated with this disorder. BAL macrophages from rheumatoid-arthritis patients without signs of ILD spontaneously release almost ten times as much superoxide as those of controls; the PMA-triggered O_2^--generation is twice that of controls (Perez et al., 1989).

The latex stimulation-induced lucigenin-enhanced chemi-luminescence of alveolar macrophages from asthmatic individuals is increased relative to that of normal individuals and is inversely correlated to the provocative dose of methacholine producing a 20 % fall in FEV_1 (Kelly et al., 1988). Alveolar macrophages from patients with allergic asthma generate more superoxide after stimulation with FMLP than the corresponding cells from controls do (Damon et al., 1988).

In patients with chronic air-flow disease, there is a corre-lation between the degree of bronchial responsiveness to hista-mine and peripheral blood PMN superoxide production triggered by PMA (Postma et al., 1988).

Alveolar macrophages from rats with an acute lung injury due to a reverse passive Arthus reaction produce more superoxide radicals after challenge with PMA than cells from non-injured lungs, an observation which suggests that changes in alveolar-macrophage function may mediate and/or resolve acute inflammatory lung injury (Brieland et al., 1987). Alveolar macrophages from patients with systemic lupus erythematosus (SLE) do not differ from those of normal individuals with respect to PMA- or STZ-triggered chemiluminescence responses (Wallaert et al., 1987).

CONCLUSION: The oxidative response of airway phagocytes is probably an important variable to follow in the characterization of various forms of inflammation in relation to airway disease.

DISCUSSION

Widdicombe.   How do steroids influence the processes you have described?

Bergstrand.   As far as we know from the literature and from own experience, GCS treatment has a surprisingly small influence on phagocyte oxidative responses, either if assessed after treating cells with corticosteroids in vitro or after treating individuals in vivo and examining cells ex vivo.

Stockley.   We have recently studied the effect of oral steroid therapy on neutrophil function in healthy subjects. The therapy had no effect on spontaneous PMA stimulated superoxide production. I think that GCS treatments have differential effects on various neutrophil functions.

Bergstrand.   I fully agree with you and I think you find ample evidence for that in the literature.

Chung.   But _in vitro_ corticosteroids can inhibit the release of

superoxide anions from human alveolar macrophage and human
eosinophils stimulated by opsonized zymosan (our own data).

Laitinen.   Has N-acetylcystein or vitamin E effect on the
oxidative burst?

Bergstrand.   If they have, I would think that it is more likely
that they act as scavengers rather than by inhibiting the
generation of reactive oxygen derived metabolites, e.g. N-
acetylcystein was recently shown to act as a hydroxyl radical
scavenger.

REFERENCES

Babior, B.M. (1987) TIBS, June, 241-243.
Babior, B.M. (1988) Arch. Biochem. Biophys. 264, 361-367.
Bass, D.A., McPhail, L.C., Schmitt, J.D., Morris-Natschke, S.,
    McCall, C.E., and Wykle, R.L. (1989) J. Biol. Chem. 264,
    19610-19617.
Bellavite, P. (1988) Free Radic. Biol. Med. 4, 225-261.
Bergstrand, H., Björnson, A., Eklund, A., Hernbrand, R., Larsson,
    K., Linden, M., and Nilsson, A. (1986) J. Free Radic. Biol.
    Med. 2, 119-127.
Berton, G., Dusi, S., Serra, M.C., Bellavite, P., and Rossi, P.
    (1989) J. Biol. Chem. 264, 5564-5568.
Borregaard, N. (1988) Eur. J. Haematol. 41, 401-413.
Brieland, J.K., Kunkel, R.G., and Fantone, J.C. (1987) Am. Rev.
    Respir. Dis. 135, 1300-1306.
Calhoun, W.J., Salisbury, S.M., Chosy, L.W., and Busse, W.W.
    (1988) J. Lab. Clin. Med. 112, 147-156.
Cantin, A.M., North, S.L., Fells, G.A., Hubbard, R.C., and
    Crystal, R.G. (1987) J. Clin. Invest. 79, 1665-1673.
Cantin, A., Dubois, F., and Bégin, R. (1988) J. Leukocyte
    Biol. 43, 299-303.
Clement, A., Chadelat, K., Masliah, J., Housset, B., Sardet, A.,
    Grimfeld, A., and Tournier, G. (1987) Am. Rev. Respir. Dis.
    136, 1424-1428.
Cooper Jr, J.A.D., Merrill, W.W., Rankin, J.A., Sibille, Y., and
    Buck, M.G. (1988) J. Appl. Physiol. 64, 1615-1623.
Curnutte, J.T., Scott, P.J., and Mayo, L.A. (1989) Proc. Natl.
    Acad. Sci. USA 86, 825-829.
Damon, M., Vial, H., Crastes de Paulet, A., and Godard, P. (1988)
    FEBS Lett. 239, 169-173.
Ding, A.H., and Nathan, C.F. (1987) J. Immunol. 139, 1971-1979.
Edwards III, C.K., Ghiasuddin, S.M., Schepper, J.M., Yunger,

L.M., and Kelley, K.W. (1988) Science <u>239</u>, 769-771.

Fels, A.O.S., Nathan, C.F., and Cohn, Z.A. (1987) J. Clin. Invest. <u>80</u>, 381-386.

Hubbard, R.C., Ogushi, F., Fells, G.A., Cantin, A.M., Jallat, S., Courtney, M., and Crystal, R.G. (1987) J. Clin. Invest. <u>80</u>, 1289-1295.

Kelly, C., Ward, C., Stenton, C.S., Bird, G., Hendrick, D.J., and Walters, E.H. (1988) Thorax <u>43</u>, 684-692.

Koenderman, L., Yazdanbakhsh, M., Roos, D., and Verhoeven, A.J. (1989) J. Immunol. <u>142</u>, 623-628.

Koren, H.S., Devlin, R.B., Graham, D.E., Mann, R., McGee, M.P., Horstman, D.H., Kozumbo, W.J., Becker, S., House, D.E., McDonnell, W.F., and Bromberg, P.A. (1989) Am. Rev. Respir. Dis. <u>139</u>, 407-415.

Marcy, T.W., and Merrill, W.W. (1987) Clinics in Chest Medicine <u>8</u>, 381-391.

Naccache, P.H., Therrien, S., Caon, A.C., Liao, N., Gilbert, C., and McColl, S.R. (1989) J. Immunol. <u>142</u>, 2438-2444.

Nathan, C.F. (1987) J. Clin. Invest. <u>80</u>, 1550-1560.

Nathan, C. F. (1989) Blood <u>73</u>, 301-306.

Nishizuka, Y. (1988) Nature <u>334</u>, 661-665.

Olsson, H., and Bergstrand, H. (1989) Cellular Signalling <u>1</u>, 405-410.

Perez, T., Farre, J.M., Goset, P., Wallaert, B., Duquesnoy, B., Voisin, C., Delcambre, B., and Tonnel, A.B. (1989) Eur. Resp. J. <u>2</u>, 7-13.

Postma, D.S., Renkema, T.E.J., Noordhoek, J.A., Faber, H., Sluiter,H.J., and Kauffman, H. (1988) Am. Rev. Respir. Dis. <u>137</u>, 57-61.

Rellstab, P., and Schaffner, A. (1989) J. Immunol. <u>142</u>, 2813-2820.

Richter, A.M., Abboud, R.T., Johal, S.S., and Fera, T.A. Lung <u>164</u>, 233-242.

Rom, W.N., Bitterman, P.B., Rennard, S.I., Cantin, A., and Crystal, R.G. (1987) Am. Rev. Respir. Dis. <u>136</u>, 1429-1434.

Rossi, F. (1986) Biochim. Biophys. Acta <u>853</u>, 65-89.

Rossi, F. Della Bianca, V., Grzeskowiak, M., and Bazzoni, F. (1989) J. Immunol. <u>142</u>, 1652-1160.

Ryer-Powder, J.E., Amoruso, M.A., Czerniecki, B., Witz, G., and Goldstein, B.D. (1988) Am. Rev. Respir. Dis. <u>138</u>, 1129-1133.

Segal, A.W. (1989) J. Clin. Invest. <u>83</u>, 1705-1793.

Sherman, M.P., and Lehrer, R.I. (1984) J. Leukocyte Biol. <u>36</u>, 39-50.

Smith, R.M., Curnutte, J.T., and Babior, B.M. (1989) J. Biol. Chem. <u>264</u>, 1958-1962.

Sullivan, R., Fredette, J.-P., Griffin, J.D., Leavitt, J.L., Simons, E.R., and Melnick, D.A. (1989) J. Biol. Chem. <u>264</u>, 6302-6309.

Wallaert, B., Aerts, C., Bart, F., Hatron, P.-Y., Dracon, M., Tonnel, A.-B., and Voisin, C. (1987) Am. Rev. Respir. Dis. <u>136</u>, 293-297.

Weiss, S.J. (1989) New Engl. J. Med. <u>320</u>, 365-376.

16) INFLAMMATORY INDICES IN CHRONIC BRONCHITIS. MONOCYTE-MACROPHAGE MICROBICIDAL ACTIVITY.

H. Nielsen

Department of Clinical Microbiology, Statens Seruminstitut, Rigshospitalet, Copenhagen 2200 N, Denmark

SUMMARY: Alveolar macrophages are important to the host defence of the lower airways. In smokers and patients with chronic bronchitis, important defects of blood monocyte functions have been identified, which may explain the increased incidence of pulmonary infections in these patients. Upon chronic stimulation, e.g. from tobacco smoke, disease may progress and macrophage activity is probably involved in the tissue damage of chronic bronchitis. As regards microbicidal activity of macrophages in patients with chronic bronchitis, no studies are available. Following pharmacological intervention, it is probably more reliable to measure specific components of macrophage metabolic and secretory activities, which are associated with microbicidal events, than to assess over-all microbicidal activity.

Phagocyte function is crucial for the host defense against invading microorganisms and this applies to the lower airways as well. The clearance of inhaled bacteria is chiefly attributed to alveolar macrophages (Green & Kass, 1964; Green & Carolin, 1967; Thomas et al., 1978; Huber et al., 1977; Pennington et al., 1984). Under normal circumstances these cells together with other lung defense mechanisms (mucociliary clearance etc.) are sufficient in keeping the lower airways sterile. The exposure to chronic smoking is the major factor in the development of chronic bronchitis, a disease characterized by repeated bacterial infections and general damage to the structure of the lung tissue due to chronic inflammation. This gives rise to increased mucus production and obstructive lung disease, which seems to progress to respiratory failure irrespectively of pharmacological treatment. However, with the better understanding of tissue damage induced by chronic inflammatory reactions, it is possible that intervention by specific anti-inflammatory agents may change the clinical course of chronic bronchitis. Thus, in the experimental therapy of chronic bronchitis with new drugs there is a need for assessment of alterations in relevant immune parameters important for disease progression.

Current research interest focuses on inflammatory cells obtained by bronchoalveolar lavage (BAL). The alveolar macrophages constitute an important part of BAL cells, in healthy subjects above 90 percent (Harris et al., 1970). In smokers the yield of alveolar macrophages is much higher than in nonsmokers (Harris et al., 1970; Mann et al., 1971). In addition, neutrophils are increased in number. Hitherto, only very few studies have evaluated the functions of BAL macrophages in patients with chronic bronchitis (as discussed elsewhere in this book), and none of these included assays of microbicidal activity. It is therefore difficult to predict the potential role of alveolar macrophage microbicidal activity as a marker in drug intervention studies. Following microbicidal challenge, macrophages release several products of potential importance for the chronic inflammatory process, i.e. toxic oxygen radicals and proteolytic enzymes. It is possible that direct measurements of these components are more reliable for the evaluation of pharmacological intervention than over-all investigations of microbidical activity. This would imply both measurement of soluble products in BAL and measurement of macrophage production of oxygen radicals in vitro immediately after bronchoscopy.

As chronic bronchitis is closely associated with smoking it is relevant to notice alterations in smokers compared with non-smokers. Blood monocytes are the precursors of tissue macrophages, and the monocytosis reported in smokers (Nielsen, 1985) is probably adaptive changes to increased recruitment of cells into the alveoli. Microbicidal activity of blood monocytes was significantly lower in otherwise asymptomatic smokers than in nonsmokers (Nielsen, 1985), but equally suppressed in smokers and chronic bronchitis patients (Nielsen & Bonde, 1986a). Since blood monocytes are the precursors of alveolar macrophages this decreased activity of the myeloperoxidase-H_2O_2-halide system in monocytes might explain, that individuals exposed to cigarette smoke have impaired pulmonary clearance of infectious organisms due to inhibition of the bactericidal activity (Green & Carolin, 1967; Spurgash et al., 1968; Rylander, 1971; Thomas et al., 1978). Nonspecific activation of monocytes/macrophages is possible with several bacterial components and products, including an extract from Klebsiella pneumonia (Nielsen, 1986), and a randomized, double-blind clinical trial with this glycoprotein extract found significant improvement in monocyte function in chronic bronchitis patients (Nielsen & Bonde, 1986b).

Interestingly, defective monocyte chemotaxis is very strongly associated with recurrent acute exacerbations in chronic bronchitis patients with hypersecretory symptoms compared with patients with obstructive symptoms only (Nielsen & Bonde, 1986a). The decreased response was equally expressed towards different cytotaxins and comprised spontaneous migratory capacity as well as directed chemotactic locomotion. An intrinsic defect of blood monocytes was suggested to explain the findings although the mechanisms were unknown. As noted above, no reports are available concerning the microbicidal activity of alveolar macrophages in chronic bronchitis.

Nevertheless, several experimental models have evaluated the influence of chronic smoking in animals, which have relevance for chronic bronchitis immunopathology. The main conclusion of such studies is that smoking is followed by impaired bactericidal clearance (Green & Kass, 1964; Rylander, 1971; Thomas et al., 1978), although other authors have failed to reproduce this (Spurgash et al., 1968; Huber et al., 1977). More selective in

vitro assays have additionally tried to measure the influence of
tobacco smoke and of components hereof on phagocyte functions.
Contradictory results have been obtained, and the experimental
models are often far from the clinical relevant situation.
However, in the study by Bridges et al. (1977) an interesting
observation was made that cysteine could prevent many of the
tobacco effects in vitro suggesting that oxidants and/or thiol-
reactive substances are involved in the inflammatory process. No
reports on macrophage microbicidal activity after cysteine
administration in patients with chronic bronchitis are available,
but could be one of several areas of clinical research in the
future.

CONCLUSION: Microbicidal activity of alveolar macrophages is
crucial for the host defense of the lower airways, but in vitro
measurement of macrophage microbicidal activity is probably less
suitable for the assessment of immunological alterations following pharmacological intervention in chronic bronchitis. Other
more specific assays should be employed. The association of
defective blood monocyte microbicidal activity in smokers and
decreased migratory capacity in chronic bronchitis with recurrent
acute exacerbations may reflect immunological disturbances
relevant to the pulmonary resistance to infections and pharmacological modulation hereof could eventually influence the
clinical course.

DISCUSSION

Hogg. What do older studies tell us on microbicidal effects?

Nielsen. Microbicidal activity has previously been studied in
several animal models, but with different conclusions! Both
impaired lung clearance of inhaled bacteria and increased
macrophage bactericidal activity in vitro have been reported

after exposure to tobacco smoke. The clinical relevance of these studies is difficult to assess. However, blood monocyte studies may be worthwhile, e.g. smokers have decreased candidacidal activity.

Stockley. I think the method you describe is interesting but I don't know if it would be useful to assess the effect of intervention. I think we need to think about two major points. Firstly, to assess intervention it is sensible at this stage to use proven and well validated methods rather than the potentially interesting ones we have heard about during this meeting. Secondly, I think we should remember that most of these tests are <u>markers</u> for inflammation and may tell us very little about the pathogenesis of conditions that may be localized to the interstitial space or submucosa. Secretion and blood studies will not necessarily reflect this process.

Nielsen. I agree that we know very little at present. Nevertheless, clinical studies are justified to create better understanding of these diseases. I believe that several assays described at this meeting are candidates as immune markers in intervention studies, but microbicidal assays are not suitable.

REFERENCES

Bridges, R.B., Kraal, J.H., Huang, L.J.T., and Chancellor, M.B. (1977) Infect. Immun. <u>15</u>, 115-123.
Green, G.M., and Carolin, D. (1967) N. Engl. J. Med. <u>276</u>, 427.
Green, G.M., and Kass, E.H. (1964) J. Clin. Invest. <u>43</u>, 769-776.
Harris, J.O., Swenson, E.W., and Johnson, J.E. (1970) J. Clin. Invest. <u>49</u>, 2086-2096.
Huber, G.L., Pochay, V.E., Mahajan, V.K., McCarthy. C.R., Hinds, W.C., Davies, P., Drath, D.B., and Sornberger, G.C. (1977) Bull. Eur. Physiopathol. Respir. <u>13</u>, 145-156.
Mann, P., Cohen, A., Finley, T., and Ladman, A (1971) Lab. Invest. <u>25</u>, 111-120.
Nielsen, H. (1985) Eur. J. Respir. Dis. <u>66</u>, 327-332.
Nielsen, H. (1986) Eur. J. Clin. Pharmacol. <u>30</u>, 99-104.
Nielsen, H., and Bonde, J. (1986a) Eur. J. Respir. Dis. <u>68</u>, 200-206.

Nielsen, H. and Bonde, J. (1986b) Int. J. Immunopharm. <u>8</u>,
    589-592.
Pennington, J.E., Ehrie, M.G., and Hickey, W.F. (1984) Rev.
    Infect. Dis. <u>6</u> (Suppl 3), 657-666.
Rylander, R. (1971) Arch. Environ. Health. <u>23</u>, 321-326.
Spurgash, A., Ehrlich, R., and Petzold, R. (1968) Arch. Environ.
    Health <u>16</u>, 385-391.
Thomas, W.R., Holt, P.G., and Keast, D. (1978) Infect. Immun. <u>20</u>,
    468-475.

17) INDICES OF INFLAMMATORY ACTIVITY IN CB AND COAD. PHAGOCYTE SECRETION AND CHEMOTAXIS.

P. Venge and Lena Håkansson

Laboratory for Inflammation Research, Department of Clinical Chemistry, University Hospital, S-751 85 Uppsala, Sweden

SUMMARY: The monitoring of inflammatory activity in the lungs of patients with chronic obstructive airways disease may be accomplished by the measurement of specific markers of inflammatory cell activity such as the eosinophil cationic protein and the neutrophil-derived myeloperoxidase. However, no specific marker, which reflects the activity of the alveolar macrophage, is available. Eosinophil and neutrophil chemotactic activity may be detected in broncho-alveolar fluid as a sign of macrophage activity. We report preliminary data, which indicate that both chemotactic activities are elevated in patients with chronic bronchitis. The predominant activities elute at a molecular weight of about 10 kDa but also at a position after the total volume of the column. We conclude that secretory products from inflammatory cells may be measured in broncho-alveolar fluid from patients with chronic bronchitis. Whether such measurements will prove useful in relation to therapeutic trials in these patients is not known but is most likely.

INTRODUCTION

The secretion of preformed granule components, and the capacity to migrate and accumulate in tissue, are two fundamental properties of phagocytic cells such as monocytes/macrophages and neutrophils. As these cells are two of the major actors in chronic bronchitis, the measuring of these activities may be expected to be helpful in the monitoring of the disease activity. As is indicated in chapter 8, the migratory activity of blood neutrophils in chronic bronchitis is raised, but only during periods with a high incidence of infectious exacerbations. The secretory activity of blood neutrophils and monocytes was only measured indirectly by means of measuring the serum levels of lactoferrin and myeloperoxidase, as indicators of neutrophil secretory activity, and of lysozyme as an indicator of monocyte/ macrophage activity. All three granule proteins were raised in patients with chronic bronchitis, indicating increased activity of the cells. However, lactoferrin and myeloperoxidase seemed to vary in accordance with the infectious exacerbations of the patients, whereas lysozyme was unaffected by these exacerbations and remained very constant throughout an observation period of 6 months. Whether any of these blood variables will be helpful in the monitoring of chronic bronchitis during a therapeutical trial is, however, not known. In this chapter, the discussion will be restricted to results obtained from the study of the secretory activity of phagocytic cells in broncho-alveolar lavage fluid (BAL) and the generation of chemotactic signals in the lung as indices of inflammatory activity in chronic bronchitis.

PHAGOCYTE SECRETION IN THE LUNG

Table I shows some proteins which have been used as indicators of phagocytic cell activity in BAL. The eosinophil has been monitored by means of its secretory products ECP, EPX/EDN or MBP and almost exclusively in relation to asthma. The specificity of these three proteins as markers of eosinophil activity varies (Dahl et al., 1988). Thus, MBP is also located in basophils (Ackerman et al., 1983). ECP and probably EPX/EDN seem to be located in eosinophils only, which makes these proteins prime candidates as specific eosinophil markers. Lactoferrin, which may be used as a specific marker of neutrophils in blood, seems to be unsuitable in this respect with regard to BAL, as it is also produced locally in the lung by glands (Reiter, 1983). This is also the case with lysozyme (Bowes & Corrin, 1977), which hampers its use as a local marker of the activity of alveolar macrophages. Myeloperoxidase, on the other hand, may be a useful marker of the local activity of neutrophils.

Table I: Some cell markers in broncho-alveolar fluid

Marker	Cellular origin
Eosinophil cationic protein (ECP)	Eosinophil
Eosinophil protein-x/Eosinophil neurotoxin (EPX/EDN)	Eosinophil derived Neutrophil?
Major basic protein (MBP)	Eosinophil Basophil
Elastase	Neutrophil
Myeloperoxidase (MPO)	Neutrophil
Lysozyme	Alveolar macrophage Submucosal glands Neutrophils
Lactoferrin	Submucosal glands Neutrophils

In a recent study, we thus found a good correlation between the number of neutrophils in BAL and the MPO concentration (Schmekel et al., 1989). Furthermore, when we collected the BAL cells - which are dominated by the presence of alveolar macrophages - and measured the MPO content in extracts from these cells, the results were well correlated to the number of neutrophils in the extract. This result suggested that the only location of MPO among BAL cells is the neutrophil. In order to substantiate this further, immunohistochemical staining of BAL cells and lung-tissue sections was performed with the aid of an antibody to MPO. These studies revealed that two cells stained with the antibody, the neutrophil and the macrophage. However, the staining of the macrophages was generally weak, and only an

average 6 % of the macrophages were stained at all, in contrast
to all neutrophils. In spite of the fact that blood monocytes do
contain MPO, they hence seem to lose this protein when they are
transformed into macrophages. The fact that a few macrophages
actually contained some MPO could be due to the active uptake of
MPO from the environment, not to true production by the cell.
Those positively stained cells could conceivably also represent
newly-recruited blood monocytes. By way of conclusion, we might
say that we probably possess good markers for the eosinophil and
the neutrophil, whereas no good marker for alveolar macrophages
has as yet been identified. However, as is shown below, the
measuring of chemotactic products in BAL may be a step in this
latter direction.

Only few studies have so far been completed, in which these
markers have been used to assess inflammatory activity in the
lung in chronic bronchitis. One study which approached this
question was performed on a group of otherwise healthy smokers,
who were given N-acetyl cysteine (NAC) in an attempt to reduce
the local consequences of smoke - i.e. the induction of an
increased inflammatory activity (Eklund et al., 1988). BAL was
performed twice, once before treatment and once after an 8-week
peroral treatment with NAC 200 mg t.i.d. Both ECP and lactoferrin
showed significant reductions after NAC treatment, whereas
lysozyme and MPO showed a clear tendency in this direction. These
results would imply that NAC reduces the inflammatory activity in
smoking individuals, and also that the secretory activity of the
glands, as reflected by reductions in lactoferrin and lysozyme,
may be reduced. Whether NAC has a similar effect on the inflammatory activity in patients with chronic bronchitis is not yet
known. In another study, these markers were used in an investigation of smokers with and without signs of lung obstruction
(Linden et al., 1988). In this study, no differences were found
between the two groups in any respect. However, it was interesting to note that the BAL levels of myeloperoxidase in these
patients were extremely closely related to those of glutathione,
which suggests a cause-and-effect relationship between these two

variables or a common origin. In most smokers, glutathione is raised in the lung fluid, and it is believed to protect the lung against the smoke-induced injurious oxygen radicals. The role of myeloperoxidase is unclear, but in the presence of a peroxide it may be one of the injurious principles.

THE GENERATION AND IDENTIFICATION OF CHEMOTACTIC ACTIVITIES IN THE LUNG

Accumulation of phagocytic cells in the lungs as a result of the recruitment of cells from the blood stream occurs by way of the adhesion of phagocytic cells to endothelial cells and the subsequent migration of cells into the lung tissue. The migration of the cells into the lungs is assumed to be mediated by the attraction of the cells by chemotactic factors. The production of chemotactic factors in lungs can be studied by means of measuring chemotactic activity in BAL fluid. Previous studies have demonstrated the presence of neutrophil and eosinophil chemotactic activity in BAL fluid from healthy individuals, smokers and non-smokers, and from asthmatic patients (Wieslander et al., 1987; Rak et al., 1988). BAL fluid from asthmatic patients obtained during a natural allergen challenge - i.e., the birch-pollen season - demonstrated increased eosinophil and neutrophil chemotactic activity. Preliminary results from a study on the chemotactic activity in BAL fluid from patients with chronic bronchitis, shown in Figure 1, demonstrated raised neutrophil and eosinophil chemotactic activity in BAL from the patients as compared with that found in healthy smokers and non-smokers. A partial characterization by means of gelfiltration of the chemotactic factors in BAL from one patient with chronic bronchitis and five healthy individuals is demonstrated in Figure 2. BAL from the chronic-bronchitis patient demonstrated several peaks of chemotactic activity. One peak which appeared in the void volume (>600 kD) and three peaks which were retarded on the column only appeared in the chromatogram of BAL from the patient. Peaks of

chemotactic activity of around 300 kD, 40-70 kD and around 10 kD
apparent molecular weight were demonstrated in both chromato-
grams, but the activity was higher in BAL obtained from the
chronic-bronchitis patient.

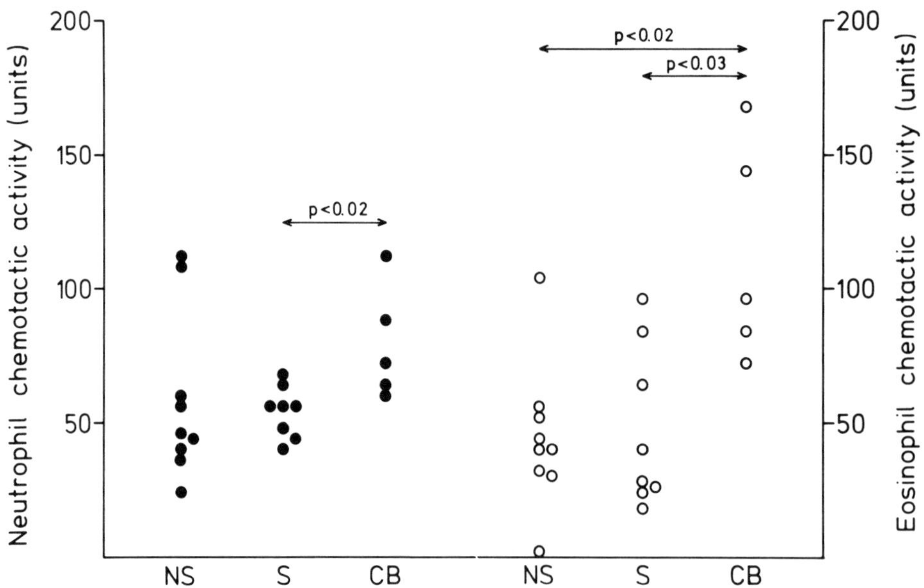

Figure 1. The neutrophil (closed circles) and eosinophil
(open circles) chemotactic activity in BAL fluid from healthy
non-smokers (NS), smokers (S) and patients with chronic
bronchitis (CB). The chemotactic activity of the samples was
evaluated from serial dilutions of the BAL fluids to detect the
maximal response of normal neutrophils and eosinophils to the
respective samples. The given chemotactic activity (units) is the
maximal chemotactic response (um) multiplied by the actual
dilution factor. The Mann-Whitney test was used in the
statistical evaluation.

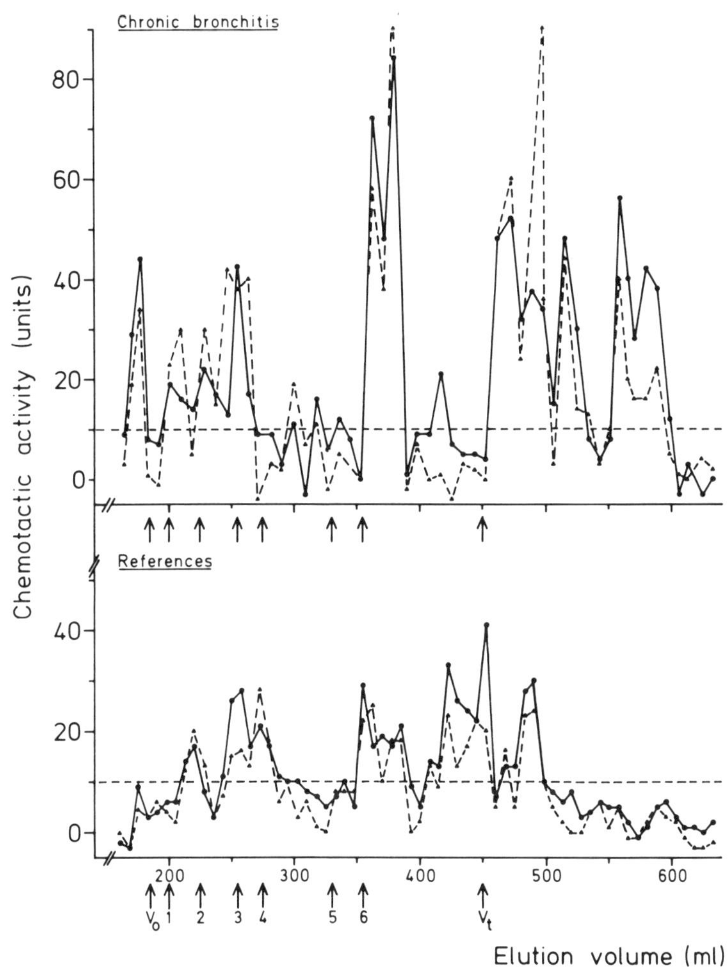

Figure 2. Gelfiltration on Sephacryl S-200 of BAL fluid from one patient with chronic bronchitis and five healthy non-smokers. The circles represent the neutrophil chemotactic activity and the triangles the eosinophil chemotactic activity. The dotted horizontal line represents the upper limit of variation of the migration towards the elution buffer (=0). The arrows indicate the elution volume of the reference proteins: 1: 440 kD, 2: 232 kD, 3: 67 kD, 4: 43 kD, 5: 25 kD and 6: 13.7 kD.

One of the possible sources of chemotactic activity obtained in BAL is the alveolar macrophage. The production of chemotactic factors by alveolar macrophages can be determined in supernatants from cultured alveolar macrophages obtained from BAL. Determination of the chemotactic activity in supernatants from healthy individuals demonstrated that the activity was markedly increased when the macrophages were stimulated with opsonized zymosan (Wieslander et al., 1987). Alveolar macrophages are able to produce LTB_4, which acts as a chemotactic factor for neutrophils and eosinophils (Palmblad et al., 1981). LTB_4 was shown to be present in BAL and in culture medium from stimulated alveolar macrophages obtained from healthy non-smokers (Wieslander et al., 1987). Furthermore, gelfiltration of culture medium from alveolar macrophages demonstrated low molecular-weight peaks of chemotactic activity, which was partly inhibited by anti-LTB_4. However, the LTB_4 concentration in BAL and culture medium from alveolar macrophages obtained from smokers was decreased as compared with that found in non-smokers, but the chemotactic activity of the samples did not show any difference between smokers and non-smokers. These results indicate that LTB_4 is one of the factors which contribute to the chemotactic activity detected in culture medium from the alveolar macrophages of non-smokers, but that in alveolar macrophages from smokers the production of LTB_4 is replaced by other chemotactic factors.

CONCLUSION: It is concluded that secretory products from inflammatory cells and chemotactic activities may be measured in broncho-alveolar lavage fluid as indicators of inflammatory activity in chronic bronchitis. Whether investigations of these activities will be useful in the monitoring of inflammatory activity in relation to therapeutic trials, is not yet known, but it seems likely.

DISCUSSION

Dahl. Could an external factor like smoking account for the decrease in e.g. MPO in BAL during the study, or can this solely be looked upon as a seasonal variation?

Eklund. As has been earlier reported today, a seasonal variation may occur in various lavage parameters. Regarding the NAC-study (Eur. Respir. J., 1988) it was performed in the period December-February and all subjects included in the study were heavy-smokers who continued to smoke to the same extent during the whole study. Thus, it does not seem plausible that the unchanged smoking habits could have influenced the MPO-content in this specific study.

Stockley. Most antisera to neutrophil elastase are predominantly directed against the active site. Thus in lavage, where the enzyme is usually bound to inhibitors, there will be reduced reactivity with the antibody. In sputum the concentrations of neutrophil elastase mirror those of myeloperoxidase and the cyto-plasmic protein L1. L1 studies were performed in collaboration with Magne Fagerhol (Oslo) and it is also present in bronchial epithelium. However, when we effectively treat patients with antibiotics the L1 concentration in sputum falls as the secretion clears (becomes mucoidal).

Laitinen. Do myeloperoxidase and tryptase in the bronchial mucosa indicate that neutrophils and mast cells have been present before?

Venge. Myeloperoxidase may be localized easily in tissues as a sign of the presence of neutrophils. I have no information on tryptase.

REFERENCES

Ackerman, S.J., Kephart, G.M., Habermann, T.M., Greipp, P.R. and
    Gleich, G.J. (1983) J. Exp. Med. 158, 946-961.
Bowes, D., and Corrin, B. (1977) Thorax 32, 163-170.
Dahl, R., Venge, P., and Fredens, K. (1988) In: Asthma, Basic
    mechanisms and clinical management, (P.J. Barnes, I. Rodger,
    and N. Thomson, Eds), Academic Press, London, pp. 115-130.
Eklund, A., Eriksson, Ö., Håkansson, L., Larsson, K., Ohlsson,
    K., Venge, P., Bergstrand, H., Björnsson, A., Brattsand, R.,
    Glennow, C., Linden, M., and Wieslander, E. (1988) Eur.
    Respir. J. 10, 832-838.
Linden, M., Håkansson, L., Ohlsson, K., Sjödin, K., Tegner, H.,
    Tunek, A., and Venge, P. (1988) Submitted for publication.
Palmblad, J., Malmsten, C.L., Uden, A.-M., Rådmark, O., Engstedt,
    L.,and Samuelsson, B. (1981) Blood 58, 658-661.
Rak, S., Björnson, A., Håkansson, L., Sörenson, S., and Venge,
    P. (1988) In: Bronchial hyperresponsiveness and cellular and
    humoral factors involved in allergic inflammation during
    pollen season. S. Rak, Dissertation from the Medical Faculty,
    University of Gothenburg, Sweden,
Reiter, B. (1983) Int. J. Tiss. Reac. 5, 87-96.
Schmekel, B., Blaschke, E., Eklund, A., Linden, M., Sundström,
    C., and Venge, P. (1989) submitted for publication.
Wieslander, E., Linden, M., Håkansson, L., Eklund, A., Blaschke,
    E., Brattsand, R., and Venge, P. (1987) Eur. J. Resp. Dis. 71,
    263-272.

AAS 30:
Inflammatory Indices
in Chronic Bronchitis
© 1990 Birkhäuser Verlag Basel

18) INFLAMMATORY INDICES FOR CHRONIC BRONCHITIS AND COAD. PROTEASES AND ANTIPROTEASES

R.A. Stockley, D. Lomas, and D. Burnett

The Lung Immunobiological Research Laboratory, The Clinical Teaching Block, The General Hospital, Steelhouse Lane, Birmingham B4 6NH, United Kingdom

SUMMARY: The study of lung secretion proteinases and their inhibitors, both functionally and quantitatively, provide information concerning the degree of inflammation in the lung. Interpretation of individual parameters may be difficult in isolation. However, a general pattern of response provides supportive evidence of a reduction in lung inflammation, including 1) reduction in plasma inhibitor concentrations, 2) increase in local inhibitor concentrations, 3) increase in enzyme inhibition, and 4) reduction in enzyme activity. Thus such changes provide an objective basis for the assessment of drug therapy.

INTRODUCTION

It is known that proteolytic enzymes can cause gross pathological changes in the lung and that deficiency of the major plasma proteinase inhibitor α-1-antitrypsin is associated with severe, early onset of emphysema (Stockley, 1983). In view of these two observations there has been rapidly expanding research into the role of proteinases and their inhibitors in the pathogenesis of chronic lung disease.

Most of the early research concentrated upon neutrophil

elastase (an enzyme known to produce experimental emphysema) and α-1-antitrypsin (because of the association of deficiency and emphysema). However, other enzymes and inhibitors have been identified over the past 20 years, many being unique to the lung and their role has yet to be clarified. Nevertheless, some of the factors which influence the presence and relationship between the enzymes and their inhibitors are becoming elucidated. It is clear from preliminary studies that inflammation and its modulation has a major influence on these proteins in the lung.

PROTEINASES

Proteolytic enzymes have been identified in sputum samples for many years, although early studies were conducted on purulent secretions. The enzymes were initially identified by their ability to digest protein substrates such as elastin, collagen and casein. More recently, the activity has been classified further as a serine, metallo or cysteine enzyme by the effect of non specific inhibitors of each class of these proteinases. In addition, peptide substrates have been developed complemented by the use of enzyme inhibitors which are highly specific for individual enzymes. Final confirmation is often obtained by the use of specific antisera.

Neutrophil Proteinases: Two neutrophil enzymes have been studied so far, although the serine proteinase neutrophil elastase (NE) has received most attention. This enzyme is preformed as the neutrophil matures in the bone marrow and the mature cell looses its ability to make the enzyme (Takahashi et al., 1988). The amount of enzyme in the cell, the numbers being recruited to the lung and the release extracellularly within the lung will all determine the local NE load.

It is not known whether therapeutic intervention can modify the NE content of the maturing neutrophils, although both steroids and non steroidal anti-inflammatory agents have been shown to modify cysteine enzyme activity in maturing monocyte-like cells (see later). However, some patients with chronic lung disease have greater neutrophil concentrations of NE (Burnett et al., 1987) although it is uncertain whether this represents cause or effect of the disease.

Recruitment of the neutrophils to the lung is a poorly understood process. It involves the release of a chemotactic signal which is "sensed" by the cell. Membrane changes increase the adherence of the cell to pulmonary endothelial cells, and the PMN then migrates "up" the chemotactic gradient. As the cell moves into the lung, it becomes activated and releases some of its NE. The process of neutrophil recruitment is usually associated with a degree of pulmonary inflammation and, as the numbers increase, with the production of purulent sputum.

Previous studies with steroids and non steroidal anti-inflammatory drugs in vitro and in animal models of inflammation have been shown to reduce the chemotactic response and subsequent inflammation. Studies in man are few and far between, although recent studies in our laboratory have shown that both types of agent have a major effect on the response of harvested neutrophils to a standard chemo-attractant in healthy subjects (Fig. 1). This observation may partly explain some of the results seen in patients receiving corticosteroid therapy (see later).

The consequences of neutrophil recruitment are seen most clearly during infective exacerbations of chronic bronchitis. Early studies had shown that NE was often detectable in secretions from patients with chronic bronchitis, although the levels rose dramatically when an infection was present (Stockley & Burnett, 1979). Furthermore, the increase during infection was in excess of the capacity of the lung inhibitors to inactivate the enzyme. Thus, free elastase activity was present during infection and has subsequently been implicated in the pathogenesis of at least the airway component of chronic lung disease (Stockley, 1987). Thus, both the quantity and activity of NE in lung secretions provides a guide to the degree of neutrophil influx and hence lung inflammation.

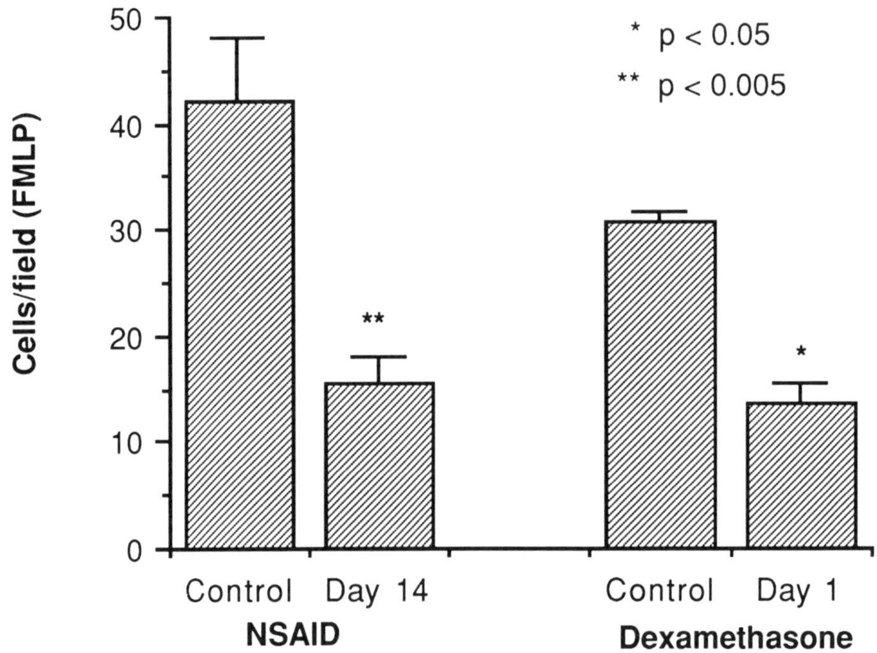

Figure 1: The effect of therapy on chemotactic response of peripheral neutrophils from healthy subjects to 10^{-8} molar FMLP. The vertical is the chemotactic response expressed as the average number of cells recruited/high power field. The histograms are mean values ± SEM for 12 subjects before and after 14 days therapy with a non-steroidal anti inflammatory agent and for 6 subjects before and on the first day of dexamethasone treatment. Significance of differences from control values are shown.

The neutrophil also contains a further serine enzyme, Cathepsin G. Studies of this enzyme in lung secretions are less advanced although its activity has been detected in purulent secretions using a specific peptide substrate (Goldstein & Doring, 1986). However, it is likely that this enzyme will be released simultaneously and thus reflect the activity of NE and provide little further information.

<u>Other Proteinases</u>: There have been very few studies of other proteinases in lung secretions, although a metallo elastase thought to be derived from bacteria has been identified in infected sputum samples (Bruce et al., 1985). Collagenolytic enzymes have been identified in lung lavage fluids, and Cathepsin B like activity has been identified in sputum. However, like all proteinases, activity depends on the amount of enzyme present and the capacity of the local inhibitors to inactivate the enzyme.

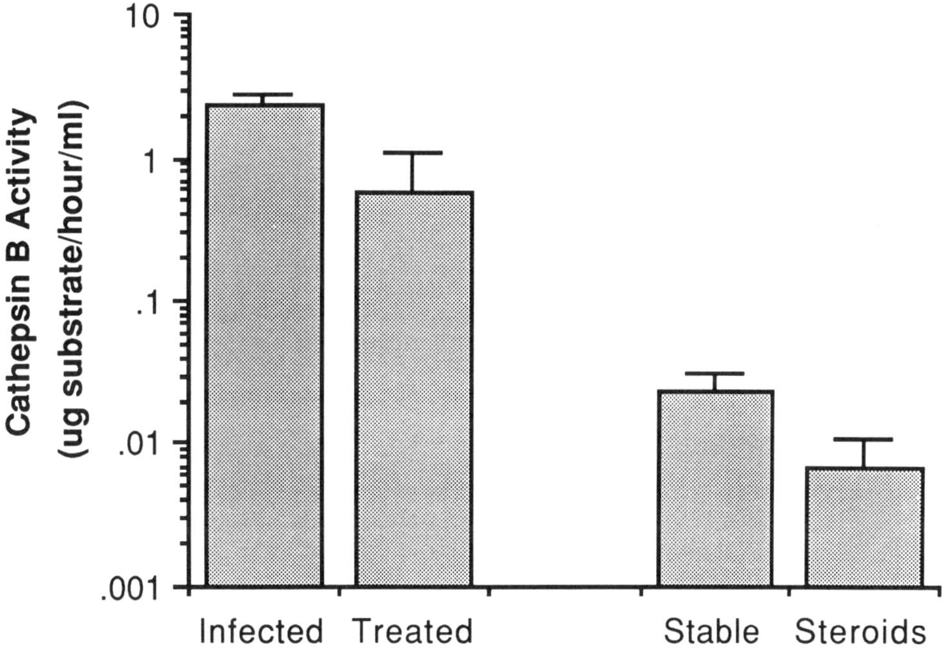

Figure 2: The effect of infection and corticosteroid therapy on lung secretion. Cathepsin B-like activity is shown expressed as units of substrate digested per ml of secretion/ hour. The details are given in the paper by Burnett & Stockley (1985).

This has been demonstrated most clearly in recent studies relating Cathepsin-B like activity to the natural inhibitors (cystatins). An inverse relationship was present, indicating that the greatest enzyme activity occurred when the cystatin C concentrations were lowest (Burnett el al., 1989). Although the source of Cathepsin-B like activity has yet to be identified, the enzyme activity undoubtedly reflects the lung inflammation and the inflammatory cell numbers in lung secretions (Burnett & Stockley, 1985). Infection increases the enzyme activity and corticosteroids reduces the activity as shown in Figure 2. Thus the secretion concentrations of this proteolytic enzyme activity may provide a good indication of the inflammatory process in chronic lung disease.

PROTEINASE INHIBITORS

It is possible to assess lung proteinase inhibitors quantitatively or by their ability to inhibit enzymes, although clearly this latter property is no longer feasible or appropriate when free activity of the target enzyme is easily detected. However, although quantitation of the inhibitor is relatively straightforward, assessment of its function may prove difficult in the presence of other inhibitors of the same enzyme.

Quantitative Studies: A variety of proteinase inhibitors have been identified in lung secretions. Some are made locally in the lung, others are solely derived by diffusion from plasma and some originate from both sources. Thus inflammation will have different effects depending upon the source of the inhibitor. Anti-leukoprotease (ALP) is a major serine proteinase inhibitor of the airway. It is produced by the serous cells of mucus glands as well as goblet cells although factors regulating its control are yet to be determined. In general terms it is believed that production of this inhibitor is fairly constant and the low concentrations found during acute infections (Fig. 3) are thought to be due to dilution of the protein as sputum volume increases (Dijkman et al., 1986). When patients receive corticosteroid therapy, the concentration of ALP increases from an average value of 20.5 mg/ml (SE ±7.7) to 39.3 ±7.4 (Stockley et al., 1986), although it is uncertain whether this indicates a reduction in sputum volume due to the steroids rather than an increase in ALP production.

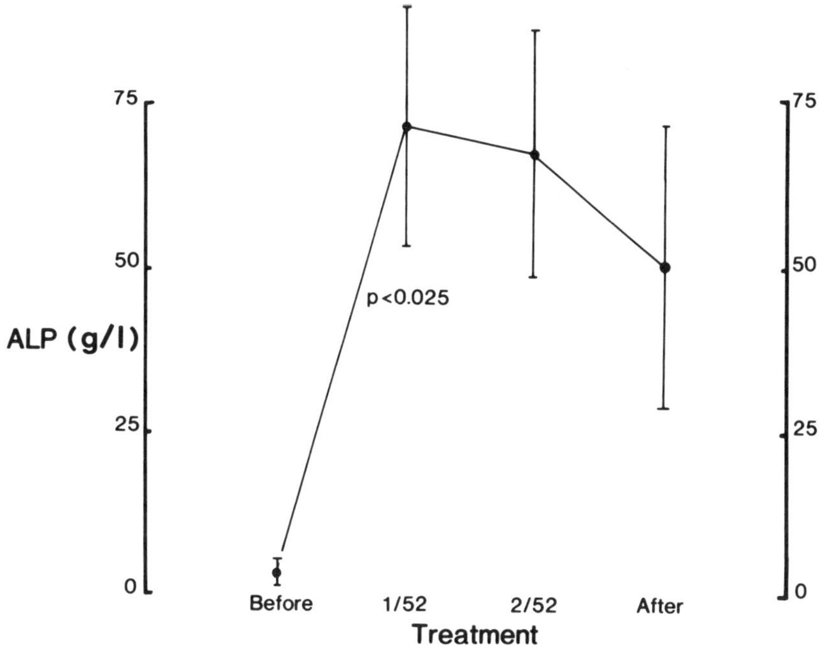

Figure 3: Sputum ALP concentration before, during and after the treatment for respiratory tract infections in patients with bronchiectasis. Mean values ± SEM are given for 10 patients. The samples were kindly assayed by J.A. Kramps, University of Leiden.

Tissue inhibitor of metalloproteinease (TIMP) functions as its name suggests and appears to be a product of the alveolar macrophage. It has been identified within lung secretions and the concentration rises with corticosteroid therapy (Burnett et al., 1986). However, although steroids can increase TIMP production by tissue fibroblasts, this may not happen with macrophages. Furthermore, the rise in TIMP concentration, like ALP, may reflect a reduction in secretion volume, although a clear anti-inflammatory effect is observed.

Studies of lung cysteine proteinase inhibitors or cystatins are even less advanced than those with TIMP. Preliminary studies show that these proteins are present, and their concentrations are related to the degree of lung inflammation as indicated by sputum purulence (Burnett et al., 1989).

The major serum derived proteinase inhibitor is α-1-anti-trypsin. The concentration of this protein in lung secretions increases in the presence of inflammation for two reasons. Firstly, the plasma concentration rises as part of the acute phase response and secondly the degree of protein "leak" from plasma increases as indicated by a rise in sputum to serum albumin ration (Stockley & Burnett, 1979).

The opposite effect is seen when patients in the stable clinical state are treated with prednisone. In this instance, the sputum and sputum/serum ratio of α-1-AT falls in a similar manner to the corresponding albumin ration (Wiggins et al., 1982). This is thought to indicate a reduction in inflammation and hence protein leakage from plasma (Wiggins et al., 1982).

Studies with the proteinase inhibitor α-1-antichymotrypsin (α-1-ACh) are more complicated. This inhibitor enters the lung from plasma as a result of protein leakage. However, in addition, a proportion of the protein appears to be produced locally in the lung (Wiggins et al., 1982). Thus there will be several factors which affect its concentrations in the lung and the association with inflammation. α-1-ACh is also an acute phase protein, and plasma concentrations rise during infection in the presence of inflammation. In addition, the degree of protein leakage from plasma increases in the presence of lung infection. Both these factors increase the concentration of α-1-ACh in the secretions. The effects of differing plasma concentrations and protein leakage are conventionally overcome by use of the secretion/plasma concentration ratios. During infection in patients with chronic bronchitis, these ratios rise from 2.56 (SE ±0.19) x 10^{-2} to 6.23 (±1.22) x 10^{-2} (Stockley & Burnett, 1980).

However, in addition there is the "local" contribution of lung cells to the secretion α-1-ACh. This contribution is usually identified by comparison with the respective albumin ratio. During the stable state the α-1-ACh ratio is on average 6.5 greater than the albumin ratio, suggesting that approximately 85 % of the sputum α-1-ACh is produced locally. During an acute chest infection, the α-1-ACh ratio rises although, because of the major effect of leakage from plasma, the ratio is only 2.1 times that of albumin, suggesting that only 52 % is made locally, i.e. the plasma contribution now approaches that of the local contribution.

Knowing the concentration of sputum α-1-ACh, it is possible to estimate the concentration being produced "locally". This rises from an average of 14.6 mg/l to 51.5 mg/l (data derived from Stockley & Burnett, 1982). This suggests a major increase in lung α-1-ACh production during infection, especially since the volume of secretion rises and hence will dilute the protein concentration more than in the stable state.

Similar precautions have to be taken in assessing lung α-1-ACh concentrations in response to anti-inflammatory therapy (steroids). In this case, the protein leakage from plasma decreases as indicated by a fall in secretion/plasma albumin ratio (Wiggins et al., 1982). The α-1-ACh ration rises from 1.38 ($\pm$0.25) x 10^{-2} to 2.57 ($\pm$0.45) x 10^{-2}. Comparison with albumin shows that the ratio is 3.5 times greater before treatment suggesting 71 % is made locally, whereas on steroid therapy, the α-1-ACh ratio is 8.5 times greater than albumin, suggesting 88 % is made locally. Again analysis of the concentrations in sputum suggest that steroid therapy raises the average value from 8.8 mg/l to 19.8 mg/l (data derived from Wiggins et al., 1982). This increase could reflect a reduction in sputum volume affecting the dilution of lung α-1-ACh, although it should be borne in mind that lung Cathepsin B actually shows a decrease in the same samples (see earlier), suggesting that any dilution affects the 2 proteins differently.

<u>Qualitative Studies</u>: The functional assessment of lung proteinases has provided to be a complex procedure. In simple terms, it should be possible to assess the ability of the secretions to inhibit a target enzyme and then relate the results to the concentration of the inhibitor present. Alternatively, when "free" enzyme activity is already present in the secretions, the implication has been that the inhibitors have been overwhelmed by excess enzyme release. Recent work from our laboratory has shown that the choice of substrate, its concentration and length of incubation as well as enzyme concentration all affect the results (Morrison et al., 1987). Even if the conditions are ideal, there are several inhibitors all of which may inactivate the target enzyme.

The simplest protein to assess is α-1-AT, as this protein appears to be the only inhibitor of porcine pancreatic elastase (PPE) in lung secretions (Morrison et al., 1986). Thus, the ability of secretions to inhibit this enzyme is solely dependent upon α-1-AT and, if the concentration is known, it is possible to assess the proportion of α-1-AT that remains functional. Many studies have shown that lung α-1-AT is largely inactive in sputum samples as a result of complexing with enzymes, oxidation and cleavage of the active site. However, in bronchitic subjects receiving corticosteroid therapy, there was no change in the ability of secretions to inhibit PPE despite the fall in α-1-AT concentration (Morrison et al., 1986). This indicated that the remaining α-1-AT was less <u>inactive</u> after steroid therapy, the proportion of inactive protein having fallen from a median value of 93 % to 89 % (data derived from Morrison et al., 1986). This is thought to reflect a reduction of α-1-AT inactivation due to partial reversal of lung inflammation and may be due to a reduction in neutrophil recruitment to the lung (perhaps reflecting the effect of steroids on chemotaxis - see Fig. 1).

Data concerning the inhibitors of neutrophil elastase (NE) is more complex, because at least 2 (α-1-AT and ALP) are present as well as a significant contribution from a third partly characterized low affinity inhibitor (Stockley et al., 1986).

Following steroid therapy, there is an increase in the ability of sputum to inhibit NE which is partly related to the increase in ALP concentrations, although the actual contribution made by this rise in inhibitor concentration is uncertain (Stockley et al., 1986).

It would be possible to obtain this information indirectly by assessing the change in NE inhibition that occurs when the ALP contribution is removed by use of an antibody. Indeed, this procedure has been successfully applied to assess the contribution of α-1-ACh to the inhibition of Cathepsin G in the presence of other effective inhibitors of this enzyme (Berman et al., 1986).

Nevertheless, it may be sufficient to quantify the total inhibitory capacity of the secretions without breaking it down into its component proteins. Certainly, an increase in collagenase inhibition also occurs on steroid therapy as the TIMP concentrations rise (Burnett et al., 1986). The general message remains the same, namely that anti-inflammatory therapy increases the enzyme inhibitory capacities of the secretions. In some instances this may reflect increases in inhibitor concentrations or a reduction in inflammatory factors which serve to inactivate the inhibitors present.

Acknowledgements: The authors thank Mrs. E.P. Ford for typing the manuscript. Many of the studies were performed whilst the authors were in receipt of funding from the MRC, British Lung Foundation, Chest, Heart and Stroke Association, West Midlands Regional Health Authority and CBHA Endowment Fund.

DISCUSSION

Hargreave. Did you measure changes in sputum volume ? How would you do it?

Stockley. Unfortunately no. This study was performed many years ago and in retrospect we should have done this. I think it would be merely a question of selecting a time period, collecting it all into a single container. This is likely to have some variability as well as all of the other measurements.

Jansen. From the studies of Kramps and your studies one can see a relation between inflammation and an increased ALP. Possibly we are dealing with a compensating process in cases of increased elastase. To my surprise, however, the NIH-group did not find changes in ALP in BAL-fluid recovered in patients with α-1-antitrypsin deficiency.

Dahl. It has been suggested that the accelerated fall in lung function is not influenced by infections. Could your findings of e.g. increased elastase and decrease of protease inhibitors during exacerbations indicate that this is of importance for the long term outcome of obstructive patients?

Stockley. Yes, it could and initially we thought that this effect would be unique to patients with chronic bronchitis and emphysema. However, similar changes occur in other patients with infections who do not have emphysema. As we discussed yesterday it remains possible that it is not the presence but the severity of the infections that may be important.

Gibson. What do your results on α_1 AT activity following corticosteroid therapy tell us about the mechanism of corticosteroid action in chronic bronchitis ?

Stockley. The fact that α-1-antitrypsin concentration falls but the inhibitory function of the protein rises, suggests that steroids affect factors which inactivate the inhibitor. This suggests that the recruitment and activation of inflammatory cells has been the primary change perhaps due to a reduction in lung secretion chemoattractants. The reduction in inflammatory cell proteinase release and superoxide production would result in an _increase_ in α-1-antitrypsin function.

REFERENCES

Berman, G., Afford, S.C., Burnett, D., and Stockley, R.A. (1986)
    J Biol. Chem., 261, 14095-14099.
Bruce, M.C., Poncz, L., Klinger, J.D., Stern, R.C., Tomashefski,
    J.F., and Dearborn, D.G. (1985) Am. Rev. Resp. Dis., 132, 529-
    535.
Burnett, D., and Stockley, R.A. (1985) Clin. Sci.,, 68, 469- 474.
Burnett, D., Reynolds, J.J., Ward, R.V., Afford, S.C., and
    Stockley, R.A. (1986) Thorax, 41, 740-745.
Burnett, D., Chamba, A., Hill, S.L. and Stockley, R.A. (1987)
    Lancet, 2, 1043-1046.
Burnett, D., Abrahamson, M., Buttle, D.J., Hill, S.L., and
    Stockley, R.A. (1989) Am. Rev. Resp. Dis., 139 (no. 4,
    part 2), A574.
Dijkman, J.H., Kramps, J.A., and Franken, C. (1986) Chest, 89,
    731-736.
Goldstein, W., and Doring, G. (1986) Am. Rev. Resp. Dis., 134,
    49-56.
Morrison, H.M., Kramps, J.A., Dijkman, J.H., and Stockley, R.A.
    (1986) Thorax, 41, 435-441.
Morrison, H.M., Kramps, J.A., Afford, S.C., Burnett, D., and
    Stockley, R.A. (1987) Clin. Chim. Acta. 162, 165-174.
Stockley, R.A. (1983) Clin. Sci. 64, 119-126.
Stockley, R.A. (1987) Clinics in Chest Medicine, 8, no. 3, 481-
    494.
Stockley, R.A., and Burnett, D. (1979) Am. Rev. Resp. Dis. 120,
    1081-1086.
Stockley, R.A., and Burnett, D. (1980) Am. Rev. Resp. Dis. 122,
    81-88.
Stockley, R.A., Morrison, H.M., Kramps, J.A., Dijkman, J.H., and
    Burnett, D. (1986) Thorax 41, 442-447.
Takahashi, H., Nukiwa, T., Basset, P., and Crystal, R.G.
    (1988) J. Biol. Chem. 263, 2543-2547.
Wiggins, J., Elliott, J.A., Stevenson, R.D., and Stockley, R.A.
    (1982) Thorax,, 37, 652-656.

19) EXUDATIVE INDICES IN AIRWAYS INFLAMMATION

C.G.A. Persson

Department of Clinical Pharmacology, University Hospital of Lund,
Lund, Sweden.

SUMMARY: Airways inflammation has come to be equated with the
presence of inflammatory cells and their products in airway lumen
and tissue. However, the inflammatory condition must also, or
rather, be determined by indices which show to what degree the
tissue itself is affected by the process. Plasma exudation from
abundant subepithelial microvessels is a specific defence/inflam-
matory tissue response to mucosal provocations; promptly after
extravasation, the plasma exudate reversibly and non-injuriously
creates intercellular pathways across the mucosa; the exudate
enters the airway lumen without compromising the epithelial
lining as a barrier to luminal solutes; there is a good correlation between surface and tissue plasma exudates. I propose that
plasma tracers on the mucosal surface can identify the ongoing
airway inflammation, its intensity and time-course in great
detail.

INTRODUCTION

Asthma and rhinitis are now defined as inflammatory diseases
largely because anti-inflammatory drugs, notably glucocorticoids,
are distinctly effective in reducing asthmatic and rhinitic
symptoms. An anti-exudative action may be a major therapeutic
effect of glucocorticoids in these diseases (Andersson & Persson,
1988; Persson & Pipkorn, 1990). Chronic bronchitis and chronic
obstructive airway disease are not equally well defined by way of

the clinical efficacy of glucocorticoids. However, retrospective studies suggest the possibility that long-term treatment with these drugs may reduce the annual decline in lung function in patients with severe and moderate to severe chronic bronchitis (Postma et al., 1985; 1988).

In 1964, Bonomo & D'Addabo demonstrated an abnormally rapid loss of intravenously injected ^{131}I-albumin into the sputum of patients with chronic bronchitis. This observation suggested that plasma exudation, as a significant sign of mucosal inflammation, was prominent in the airways of these patients. The findings of Bonomo & D'Addabo (1964) were recently confirmed (Honda et al., 1988) and interpreted as evidence of ongoing plasma exudation in the airways of these patients (Persson, 1988a).

It is not only the studies carried out with iodine-labelled albumin that suggest the occurrence of plasma exudation in chronic bronchitis. Elevated concentrations of albumin, IgG and other proteins, which would indicate the presence of exuded plasma, have also been found in sputum samples. Particularly high levels of these proteins were found in connection with exacerbations (Stockley et al., 1979; Moretti et al., 1984). However, glucocorticoid treatment reduced the sputum concentration of plasma proteins even in patients with stable chronic bronchitis (Wiggins et al., 1982).

The present discussion is concerned with the relative merits of plasma exudation as a marker of ongoing mucosal/submucosal inflammation in tracheobronchial airways.

PROINFLAMMATORY CELLS MAY NOT SHOW ONGOING INFLAMMATION

The presence of neutrophils, eosinophils, mast cells, platelets, lymphocytes, and/or basophils and select products of these cells has come to be equated with inflammation. However, the inflammatory cells may be present in the airways in order to carry out tissue repairs, or they may be there without affecting the tissue. Therefore, such cells are, not always markers of inflammation. Indeed, it is only when one can ascertain that the cells are actively fuelling an inflammatory process in the airway tissue that cell counts and cell products may define airways inflammation. Even if such a definition has been reached, the relationship between cell numbers and the degree of inflammation remains unknown. In the last few decades, a rapidly-increasing number of studies of airways inflammatory cells have been put forward, improving our knowledge of the mechanisms that may be involved in airways disease processes. As markers of inflammation, however, the cells and their products have severe limitations. Ideally, a marker of ongoing inflammatory processes should tell us to what degree the airway tissue itself is affected.

WHICH TISSUE RESPONSE IS INFLAMMATION?

Inflammation may be viewed as a misdirected and exaggerated defence reaction. But not all aspects of airway defence would qualify as specific signs of inflammation. Tracheobronchial smooth-muscle constriction, although it may be induced by an inflammatory process, is not characteristic of inflammation. Similarly, secretion may be induced by a variety of stimuli which are not necessarily inflammatory in nature. The vasodilation involved in increased blood flow and congestion explains the "rubor" of inflammation. However, this vascular effect _per se_ is not inflammation. Bronchial tone, secretions, and blood flow are all under significant neural control and are significantly affected by irritant types of provocations. The most powerful neural tracheobronchial reflex is cough but, again, cough is not exclusive to inflammation, nor is it always induced by it.

In 1882, Cohnheim wrote a famous treatise on inflammation. From his general observations on inflammation, the following can be deduced and applied to the airways (Persson 1986; 1988b): "There is no inflammation without tracheobronchial blood vessels. - The inflammatory stimulus directly affects the endothelial cells of the vessel wall to increase permeability and produce plasma exudation. - The proteinaceous exudate is a cardinal sign of inflammation. - Plasma exudation and leukocyte extravasation are distinct inflammatory events. - The plasma exudate will pass across the mucosa to mix with secretions."

The plasma-exudation response is not just an exaggeration of the normal capillary exchange of fluid and solutes. Plasma-exudation is a specific defence/inflammatory response on the part of postcapillary venules (Fig 1). Furthermore, recent observations in animal airways suggest that plasma tracers on the surface of the airway mucosa reflect ongoing inflammatory processes affecting the underlying tissue in great detail (Persson & Erjefält, 1986; Erjefält & Persson, 1989).

EXTRAVASATION OF PLASMA IS REGULATED BY ACTIVE VENULAR ENDOTHELIAL CELL SEPARATION AND HYDROSTATIC PRESSURE

Under baseline conditions, the vascular-interstitial fluid balance is maintained by the elevated hydrostatic pressure in capillary beds and by the opposing force of the transmural colloid osmotic pressure. Inflammatory effects on the vessel wall produce a dramatic change which locally abolishes the colloid osmotic-pressure gradient. The vascular target cells responsible for increased permeability to macromolecules in inflammation are the endothelial cells of the postcapillary venules (see Persson & Svensjö, 1985; Grega et al., 1988). Receptors for a variety of agents are present on these cells. Inflammatory agents, perhaps through some contractile action, actively separate the endothelial cells so as to produce gaps in the venular wall (Fig. 1). Exudation of plasma through these gaps is then brought about by the hydrostatic pressure gradient. The plasma-exudation response may also be regulated by blood flow. However, the airway mucosa/submucosa may be so well perfused with blood that pharmacologically induced changes in blood flow may not have much influence on the exudation process.

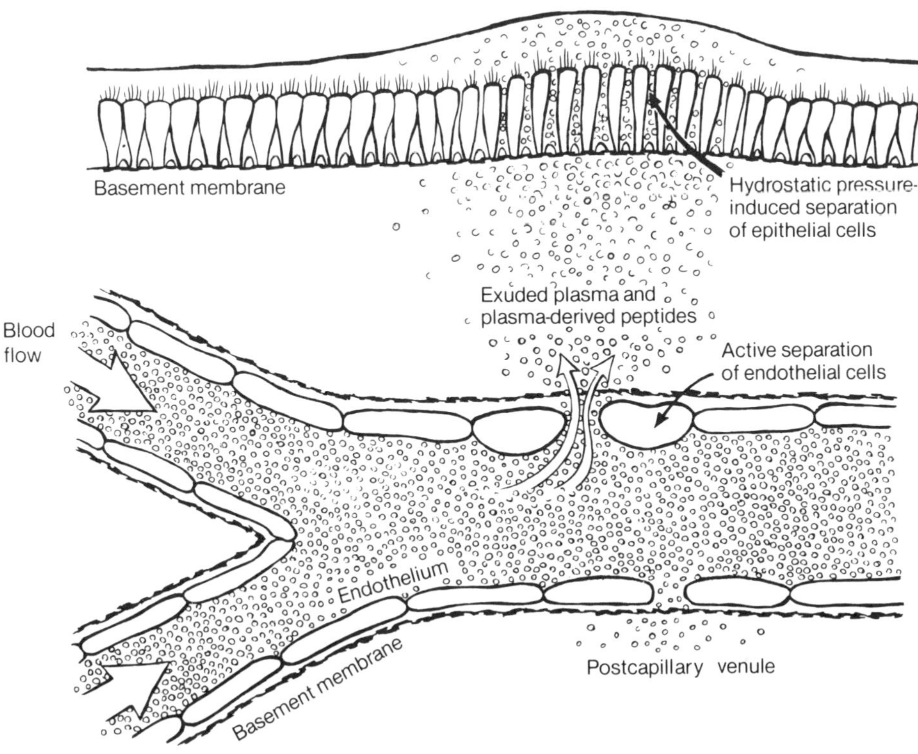

Figure 1. A proposed concept of the airways plasma exudation process is illustrated (see text).

INCREASED HYDROSTATIC PRESSURE IN THE INTEREPITHELIAL INTERSTITIAL SPACE MAY REGULATE THE PASSAGE OF PLASMA EXUDATE ACROSS THE MUCOSA

Following mucosal provocation, plasma is exuded from the abundant subepithelial microvessels (Fig. 1, 2) and distributed in the interstitial space. Since the epithelial cells are separate from the base up to the apical region, their sides would be compressed by the exudate. At a certain hydrostatic pressure, the tight

apical parts would also separate. An intercellular pathway may
thus be created through which the plasma exudate can flow into
the lumen. Such flow would be along a hydrostatic pressure
gradient; hence, it would be unidirectional (Fig. 1). When the
interstitial pressure is again reduced towards normal values,
epithelial tight junctions would be reestablished. Indeed,
promptly after the mucosal passage of a large volume of plasma
exudate, such as would more than replace the entire periciliary
fluid layer, the epithelial lining looked intact in light microscopy and electron microscopy examinations (unpublished work by
Luts, Sundler, Erjefält and Persson).

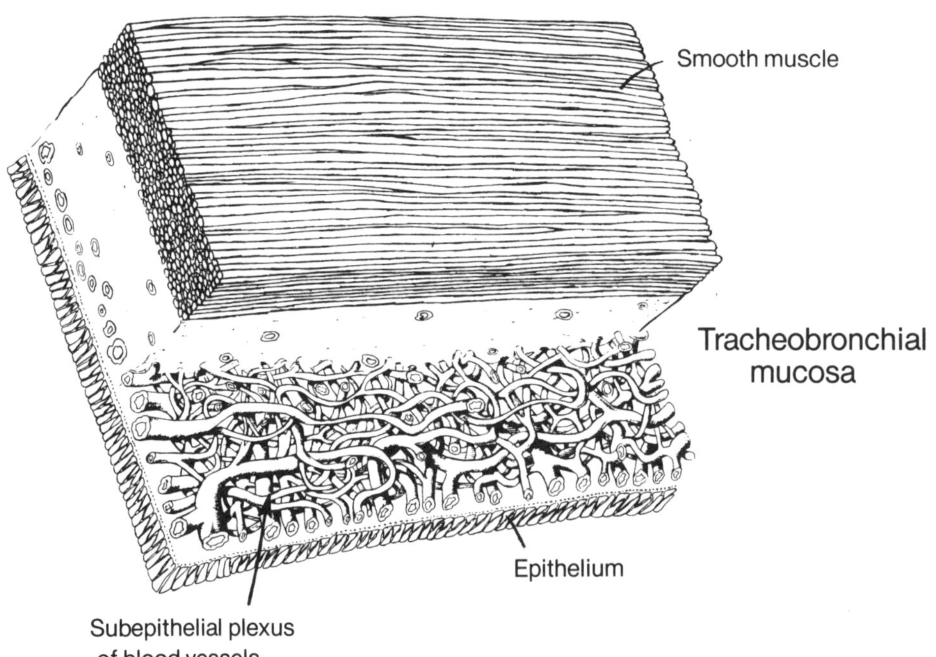

Figure 2. This schematic drawing of the tracheobronchial
wall emphasizes the abundance of microvessels just beneath the
epithelial lining.

In a recent study of guinea-pig isolated tracheal tubes, it was demonstrated that a serosal-to-mucosal hydrostatic pressure difference of only 5 cm H_2O was sufficient to produce the significant luminal entry of a serosal macromolecular tracer. Such pressure-induced epithelial responses were reversible and repeatable (Persson et al., 1990), indicating that this in-vitro mechanism of unidirectional mucosal crossing, may reflect what actually occurs during airways plasma exudation in vivo.

PLASMA EXUDATION AS A PRIMARY MUCOSAL DEFENCE MECHANISM

Mainly because the normal airway epithelium is considered to be such a tight barrier, plasma exudation has not previously been put forward as an important mucosal defence mechanism. In view of the accumulation of data on airway exudations, and in view of our increased understanding of how a plasma exudate may seep through the normal airway mucosa, this negative view may no longer be tenable (Persson, 1990).

The consistent passage of exuded plasma into the airway lumen in connection with mucosal provocations identifies the subepithelial microvessels as an integral part of the mucosal surface defence system. The exudation is largely an unfiltered flow of plasma (Persson & Erjefält, 1986; Erjefält & Persson, 1989) and would thus allow circulating immunoglobulins, as well as other potent plasma protein systems (kinin-, complement-, coagulation-, fibrinolysis- etc.), to operate on mucosal surfaces distinctly at sites where the mucosa is being attacked.

In the process of exudation, the plasma proteins come in contact with activating factors such as negatively charged surfaces. An abundance of potent plasma-derived peptides is thus being produced. The appearance of bradykinins on the mucosal surface has been particularly well documented (Baumgarten et al., 1986; Svensson et al., 1989). Newly formed peptides of the exudate will not only be potent mediators. By means of osmotic forces, these molecules will attract fluid and make the exudate/

transudate increasingly voluminous. By means of its actions and its volume, the plasma exudate will complement and cooperate with the mucociliary escalator in the defence operations of the airway surface.

As a first line of defence, it seems important that the exudation can occur without compromising the mucosa as a barrier to luminal solutes. In-vivo studies in both animal tracheobronchial airways (Erjefält & Persson, 1989) and human nasal airways (Greiff et al., 1990) have demonstrated that the absorption of macromolecules may not be increased during the acute exudation phase, when plasma tracers such as albumin, fibrinogen, and dextrans enter the lumen. This separation of exudation and absorption permeabilities may explain why there is now compelling evidence to support the contention that plasma exudation does occur in asthma, bronchitis, and rhinitis, whereas an abnormally increased mucosal absorption of airway macromolecules has not been demonstrated in these diseases (Persson 1986; 1989; Persson & Pipkorn, 1990).

Stimulus-induced plasma exudation usually goes on for a few minutes only because the mechanisms geared to closing the vascular leak are strong. Even in the continuous presence of an inflammatory mediator, a spontaneous closure takes place. Hence, in most instances the defence reaction will only be a brief localized burst of plasma exudate into the lumen.

PLASMA EXUDATION INTO THE LUMEN DEFINES ONGOING MUCOSAL/-SUBMUCOSAL INFLAMMATION

The plasma-exudation response is graded in accordance with the number of venular leaky sites and the amount of exuded plasma per unit time (Grega et al., 1988). Part of the plasma exudate will be removed by the lymphatic system. However, this appears to be a slow process compared with the prompt clearance of exudate into the airway lumen (Erjefält & Persson, 1989 and unpublished data). Hence, inflammatory mucosal provocations produce dose-related exudative responses which can equally well be detected in airway tissue and lumen. Indeed, threshold exudative effects were even more evident in samples of airway surface liquids than in the tissue (Erjefält & Persson, 1989).

Human studies of airways plasma exudation are greatly facilitated by the observation that plasma tracers in mucosal surface liquids almost immediately reflect the condition of the underlying tissue (Erjefält & Persson, 1989). Through broncho-alveolar lavage and through sampling of sputum, airway mucosal surface liquids can be obtained in human subjects. But which tracers of plasma exudation should be analyzed?

The inflammatory stimulus-induced increase in endothelial-epithelial exudation permeability is so great that little or no size-selectivity seems to remain for the luminal entry of plasma solutes. In theory, therefore, the composition of plasma proteins in the exudate, at least during the acute phase, is close to that of plasma circulating in the blood. Thus, any of the medium- to large-sized plasma proteins should supply a useful quantitative measure of the exudation.

During its passage into airway tissue and lumen and thereafter, the plasma exudate attracts fluid because of the rapid accumulation of break-down peptides. Generally, therefore, the volume of the exudate will be underestimated whenever calculations are based on macromolecular tracers. The problem of recording the actual volume of a plasma exudate/transudate has not been solved.

Albumin has been most frequently analyzed in different airway samples. Albumin is not a very large molecule, and it is the most common protein found in normal airway liquids. Albumin may also be actively secreted by the airway mucosa (Widdicombe, this volume). Particularly in bronchoalveolar-lavage liquids, albumin is not always an adequate tracer of airway plasma exudation. Firstly, this technique primarily tends to sample alveolar lining fluid (the solutes of which reflect pulmonary, and not tracheo-bronchial, endothelial-epithelial barrier functions). Secondly, what is brought up by the lavage has accumulated on the bronchoalveolar surface for an unknown period of time. Therefore, any induced changes in airway albumin levels may be obscured in the high and variable background concentrations of this particular protein.

There are means to circumvent many of the problems stated above. Specific bronchial lavages have been successful (Lam et al., 1985). Radiolabelled albumin can be injected as a plasma tracer in order to reduce and define the time period during which the exudation of this tracer is evaluated. Larger proteins may be more specific plasma tracers than albumin because very few of them would normally pass into the lumen.

LEARNING FROM THE NASAL MUCOSA

In the human nasal mucosa, airway specificity is no problem, and a low and consistent background of exudative indices is easily obtained by means of prior lavages with saline. In liquids from human nasal lavage, albumin reflects plasma exudation quite well. This is indicated by the concomitant exudation of fibrinogen and albumin, at a ratio which is similar to that present in circulating plasma (unpublished work by Alkner, Persson, Pipkorn, Svensson). The human data confirm findings previously obtained in guinea-pig tracheobronchial airways (Erjefält & Persson 1989).

Inflammatory indices which were originally thought to be cellular in origin also appear on the mucosa of the inflamed nasal airways as part of the plasma-exudation process. Thus, nasal-lavage-fluid levels of TAME-esterase activity and kinins indicate that plasma exudation occurs during inflammatory provocations in the laboratory (Baumgarten et al., 1986; Svensson et al., 1989) and during natural exposure to allergens (Andersson et al., 1989; Svensson et al., 1990).

The increasing support given to the idea that the barrier functions of nasal and tracheobronchial airways are similar, in health and in disease, is promising. Through the specific, ethical, and versatile experimental possibilities that the human nasal mucosa provides, we can learn much about the important pathophysiology and pharmacology of absorption and exudation permeabilities. The nasal studies can be matched by tracheobronchial experiments in animals, and particularly important points can then be selected for examination in human bronchi in vivo.

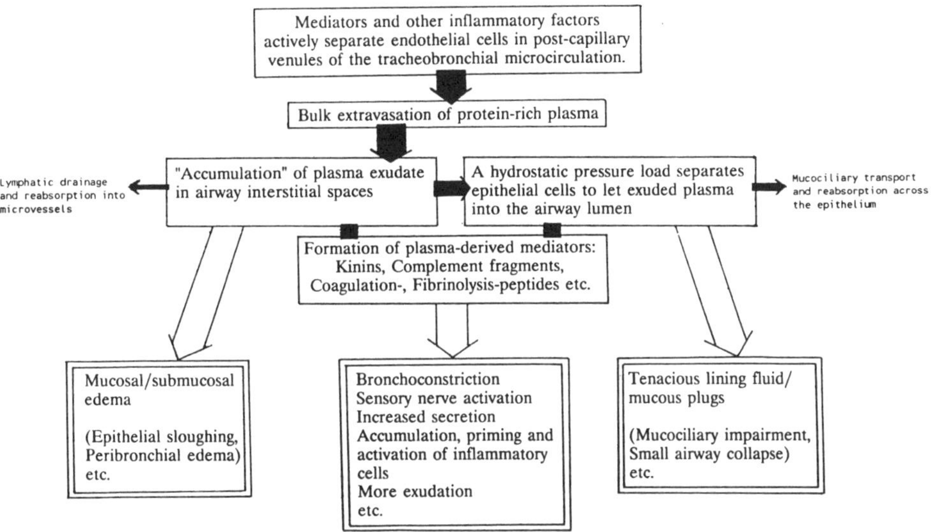

Figure 3. The center of this scheme depicts various steps in the airways plasma exudation/transudation process (black arrows). Beneath, connections with airway pathology are indicated.

EXUDED PLASMA MAY ALSO BE PATHOGENETIC

Airways plasma exudation received significant attention only a few years ago when its pharmacological regulation and, particularly, its potential pathogenetic roles were delineated (Persson 1986; 1988b). In addition to being a marker of inflammation, the exuded plasma may significantly contribute to the physical and physiological pathology of inflammatory airways disease (Fig. 3).

CONCLUSION: It is concluded that exuded plasma on the surface of an intact or damaged airway mucosa is a quantitative measure of ongoing inflammatory processes in the airways.

DISCUSSION

Jansen. When a rather massive plasma protein leakage from the submucosal microvasculature is a primary event after allergen inhalation, the endothelial cell will be the target cell. That will mean that the allergen at least should penetrate or be absorbed through the epithelium. Is there any evidence for an increased absorption of allergens in allergic asthma?

Persson. No, not that I know of. However, experimentally we have observed that the exudation/transudation of plasma is not necessarily associated with an increased absorption of luminal macromolecules.

Gibson. Is there evidence for plasma exudation in mild stable asthmatics?

Persson. Yes, I think Dr Jansen, for example, has obtained such evidence.

REFERENCES

Andersson, M., Svensson, C., Andersson, P., and Pipkorn, U. (1989) Am. Rev. Respir. Dis. _139_, 911-914.

Andersson, P., and Persson, C.G.A. (1988) In: Directions for new antiasthma drugs (S.R. O'Donnell, C.G.A. Persson, Eds.) Basel, Birkhäuser, pp 239-260.

Baumgarten, C.R., Nichols, R.C., Naclerio, R.M., Lichtenstein, L.M., Norman, P.S., and Proud, D. (1986) J. Immunol. 137, 977-982.

Bonomo, L., and D'Addabo, A. (1964) Clin. Chim. Acta 10, 214-222.

Erjefält, I., and Persson, C.G.A. (1989) Pulmonary Pharmacol. 2, 93-102.

Grega, G.J., Persson, C.G.A., and Svensjö, E. (1988) In: Endothelial cells (U.S. Ryan Ed.) CRC Press, Boca Raton, pp 103-119.

Greiff, L., Pipkorn, U., Wollmer, P., Alkner, U., and Persson, C.G.A. (1990) Eur. Respir. J. (suppl.) (in press).

Honda, J., Shimuta, S., Sasaki, T., Sasaki, H., Takishima, T., and Nakamura, M. (1988) Am. Rev. Respir. Dis. 137, 866-871.

Lam, S., Leriche, J.C., Kijeck, K., and Phillips, R.T. (1985) Chest 88, 856-859.

Moretti, M., Giannico, G., Marchioni, C.F., and Bisetti, A. (1984) Eur. J. Respir. Dis. 65, 365-370.

Persson, C.G.A. (1986) Lancet 2, 1126-1129.

Persson, C.G.A., and Erjefält, I. (1986) Acta Physiol. Scand. 126, 615-616.

Persson, C.G.A. (1988a) Am. Rev. Respir. Dis. 138, 1646-1647.

Persson, C.G.A. (1988b) Lung 166, 1-23.

Persson, C.G.A. (1989) In: Bronchitis IV (H.J. Sluiter, and R. Van der Lende, Eds.) Van Gorcum, Assen, pp 236-248.

Persson, C.G.A. (1990) Eur. Respir. J. (in press).

Persson, C.G.A., Erjefält, I., and Gustafsson, B. (1990) Int. Arch. Allergy Appl. Immunol. (in press).

Persson, C.G.A., and Pipkorn, U. (1990) In: Asthma and rhinitis. Similarities and differences. (N. Mygind, R. Dahl, U. Pipkorn, Eds.) Copenhagen, Munksgaard, pp 275-288.

Persson, C.G.A., and Svensjö, E. (1985) In: Handbook of inflammation, Vol. 5. The pharmacology of inflammation (I.L. Bonta, M.A. Bray, M.J. Parnham, Eds.) Amsterdam, Elsevier, pp 61-81.

Postma, D.S. Steenhuis, E.J., Van der Weele, L.T.H., and Sluiter, H.J. (1985) Eur. J. Respir. Dis. 67, 56-64.

Postma, D.S., Peters, I., Steenhuis, E.J., and Sluiter, H.J. (1988) Eur. Respir. J. 1, 22-26.

Stockley, R.A., Mistry, M., Bradwell, A.R., and Burnett, D. (1979) Thorax 34, 777-782.

Svensson, C., Baumgarten, C.R., Pipkorn, U., Alkner, U., and Persson, C.G.A. (1989) Thorax 44, 13-18.

Svensson, C., Andersson, M., Persson, C.G.A., Venge, P., Alkner, U., and Pipkorn, U. (1990) J. Allergy Clin. Immunol. (in press).

Wiggins, J., Elliott, J.A., Stevenson, R.D., and Stockley, R.A. (1982) Thorax 37, 652-656.

20) THE MEASURING OF "RESPIRATORY-MEMBRANE PERMEABILITY" AND LOCAL PRODUCTION OF IMMUNOGLOBULINS AND ANTIBODIES BY MEANS OF AN ANALYSIS OF SPUTUM.

E.A. van de Graaf[1,2], T.A. Out[2], and H.M. Jansen[1]

[1]Department of Pulmonology, Academic Medical Centre, Amsterdam; The Netherlands, [2]Clinical Immunology Laboratory, Academic Medical Centre, and Laboratory for Experimental and Clinical Immunology, CLB, Amsterdam, The Netherlands.

SUMMARY: When measuring the exudation of serum proteins and the local production of immunoglobulins and antibodies within the lung by means of an analysis of sputum, the permeability properties of the respiratory membrane should be taken into account. In this paper, we describe the "loss of size selectivity" that usually accompanies an increased permeability on the part of the respiratory membrane. This phenomenon enables us to measure respiratory membrane permeability independently of the sputum water content. Consequences with regard to discrimination between leakage from the circulation and/or local production of immunoglobulins and antibodies are discussed. Sequential studies which take these factors into account may provide insights into the extent of local inflammatory reactions in individual patients.

INTRODUCTION

The common denominator in respect of chronic bronchitis in Chronic Obstructive Airway Disease (COAD) is the diffuse airway narrowing which occurs as a result of an increased thickness of the airway wall due to mucosal hypervascularization, edema and inflammation, together with an accumulation of mucus caused by hypersecretion from the submucosal glands and a proliferation and contraction of the smooth-muscle tissue around the airways. The inhalation or aspiration of small amounts of toxic exogenous factors, or an invasion of small numbers of micro-organisms, will not give rise to injury or local colonization in normal airways. However, changes in local conditions, like the ones that occur in chronic bronchitis and COAD, may initiate local inflammation and impair local defence systems. In the Netherlands, the prevalence of chronic bronchitis in a random population aged 35 years and older is about 10-15 %. The incidence of bacterial broncho-pulmonary infections in that population is about 30-50 %. In addition, important factors affecting the persistence of chronic bronchitis and COAD may be the existence and a history of smoking. However, other factors may also contribute to the extent of the disease. In this report we discuss the exudation of plasma proteins and the local production of immunoglobulins and anti-bodies as entities contributing to the inflammatory processes in the airways.

MUCOSAL SERUM PROTEIN LEAKAGE

The major functional characteristics of airway inflammation are increased submucosal blood flow and microvascular permeability. This contention is supported by studies in animals, in which inflammatory mediators caused vasodilatation (Laitinen et al., 1987) and an increase in the vascular and mucosal exudation-permeability of the airways (Persson, this volume). In chronic bronchitis with COAD (Stockley 1979a; 1979b), as well as in the more acute and reversible asthmatic disease states (Out et al., 1987), this has been shown to be an important pathophysiological sign. Presumably, it is caused by an effect on the airway micro-vasculature and epithelial cells of mediators released by inflam-matory cells. We recently described, in a study of mild, non-provoked asthmatics, the occurrence of a marked increase of macromolecular leakage into recovered Bronchoalveolar Lavage Fluid (BALF) (Out et al., 1987).

In animals, the "respiratory-membrane permeability" with regard to serum proteins (exudation-permeability across airway endothelial-epithelial barriers) can be measured by calculating the concentration gradients of proteins between the serum and bronchial epithelial lining fluid (ELF) (Gorin et al. 1979; Persson & Erjefält, 1986). To measure the "respiratory-membrane permeability" in sputum, we assume that the serum proteins in sputum sol phase (SSF) derive from the epithelial lining fluid (ELF). We determined the concentration gradients of these proteins between blood and the sol phase of the recovered sputum. For this purpose, we selected proteins with different molecular masses which are not produced within the lungs. Albumin (ALB) (67KD) and ceruloplasmin (CP) (132 KD) are produced in the liver and α-2-macroglobulin (A2M) (725 KD) is not produced within the lungs (Gittlin et al., 1969). The concentration gradients are expressed in the following formula:

$$Q \text{ protein} = 1000 \times \frac{[\text{protein}] \text{ in sputum sol phase}}{[\text{protein}] \text{ in serum}}$$

The amount of a protein that enters the bronchial secretions from the blood by way of diffusion depends on molecular size and serum concentrations (Stockley et al., 1979a). Inflammation in the lung results in increased transudation of proteins from the blood (Stockley et al., 1979a; 1979b). This increased "respiratory-membrane permeability" is usually accompanied by a reduction in the size selectivity of the respiratory membrane with regard to large molecules and by a relative increase in the concentrations of these molecules in the lining fluid of the peripheral lung (Bell et al., 1981; Holter et al., 1986; Out et al., 1987) and the tracheobronchial airways (see Persson this volume).

Where the analysis of protein concentrations in SSF is concerned, a major problem is the variable sputum water content and
hence the variable dilution, in the SSF, of proteins derived from
the epithelial lining fluid (ELF). In order to overcome this
problem, we used a measure for "respiratory-membrane permeability" which is independent of the variable dilution and takes
the loss of size selectivity on the part of the "respiratory-
membrane" into account (Van de Graaf et al., 1989). We primarily
described the method in a model of BALF, but since we are dealing with the same problem in sputum, this method can be applied
to sputum sol phase as well.

The permeability of the respiratory membrane is therefore
studied by means of calculating the ratio QA2M/QCP. In this
ratio, we express the relative increase in the lining fluid of a
large protein (A2M) compared to a smaller protein (CP). Since the
variable of dilution influences the denominator and the numerator
of the ratio to the same extent, QA2M/QCP is independent of the
water content of sputum.

LOCAL PRODUCTION OF PROTEINS WITHIN THE RESPIRATORY MUCOSA

Besides the lung-specific proteins, such as the surfactant
proteins and the mucus glycoproteins which are synthesized in
the lung compartment, lactoferrin and Sc(IgA)2 are examples of
proteins which are not lung-tissue-specific but predominantly
produced locally in the mucosa (Masson et al.,1966; Bowes et al.,
1981; Goodman et al., 1981; Haimoto et al., 1984; Raphael et al.,
1989). Lactoferrin is synthesized by submucosal glands, and its
concentration in bronchial secretions may be a reflection of the
activity of the gland cells. The dimeric IgA is produced by
plasma cells restricted to the periglandular and submucosal
region of the bronchial epithelium (Rossen et al., 1968; Tourville et al., 1969) and binds to the Secretory Component (SC) on
the cell surfaces. It is actively transported over epithelial
cells, during which transport a secretory component is fixed to

it, and sc(IgA)2 then diffuses into the respiratory lining fluid. The quantification of sc(IgA)2 and lactoferrin has to be performed in absolute terms as mg/l sol-phase volume.

Immunoglobulin-producing B-cells or plasma cells have been found in very low numbers in BALF from healthy individuals (Daniele et al., 1975; Lawrence et al., 1978). The main capacity for immunoglobulin production appears to reside in these cells, located in the mucosal tissue (Soutar, 1977; Hance et al., 1988). This is true of the synthesis of IgG, IgM, dimer IgA and also of IgE. The latter, however, is present in very low concentrations when no allergic reactions are involved.

For the interpretation of results regarding such proteins as IgM, which can derive from the blood but can also be produced locally, it is important to know whether these proteins originate in airway-mucosa activated plasma cells or leak from the micro-vasculature of the lamina propria. Inflammation induces an increase of the above-mentioned leakage (Persson & Erjefält, 1986). Detailed information on the permeability of the mucosal barriers is required for discriminating between the local production of these proteins on the one hand and increased leakage from the blood on the other. We have previously shown (Van de Graaf et al., 1989; Out et al., 1990) that one cannot, when estimating the local production of immunoglobulins, use such methods as the analysis of distribution coefficients (Bell et al., 1987) or the relative coefficient of excretion relative to excretion (RCE) (Delacroix et al., 1985).

The reason for this may be the loss of molecular size selectivity on the part of the respiratory membrane that will increase the leakage of IgM into the BALF more than the leakage of a small protein such as albumin. When the local production of IgM within the lung is studied, the permeability properties of the "respiratory membrane" should be taken into account. Since IgM (900kD) has about the same molecular mass as A2M (725kD), loss of size selectivity in the "respiratory membrane" will affect the permeation of A2M and IgM to the same extent. Therefore, we compare QIgM with QA2M (Van de Graaf et al., 1988) instead of with an albumin ratio, which is the usual procedure. When QIgM/QA2M is above one, we assume that there is local production, or active transport of IgM from the systemic circulation into the bronchial lining fluid has occurred.

APPLICATION IN SPUTUM SOL PHASE

Both methods of analysis of "respiratory membrane permeability" and local production of immunoglobulins are illustrated in a 52-year-old, non-smoking female patient who was admitted to hospital because of an exacerbation of her chronic obstructive airway disease. During a 23-day-stay, the patient was treated with glucocorticoids, aminophylline and inhalation of salbutamol and acetylcystein. She recovered slowly. On day 15 after admission, another exacerbation with increased wheezing and an increase of body temperature to the subfebrile level was noted. After 23 days, the patient left the hospital in good condition. Sputum was collected during day 2, 10, 11, 15 and 16. Blood was drawn on day 2.

In Figure 1, it is shown that the QA2M/QCP ratio remained low during the first 3 days of sputum collection (0.05, 0.03 and 0.03). On day 16 and 17 after admission, the QA2M/QCP ratios were 0.18 and 0.25, respectively. This suggests an increase of "respiratory-membrane permeability" on day 16 and 17.

On admission, the patient had a local production of IgM, as the QIgM/QA2M ratio was 3.69 on day 2. On day 10 and 11, the QIgM/QA2M increased to 6.50 and 12.3, respectively. Five days later, the production of IgM had decreased again.

Although not all sputum samples are matched with serum samples, this example demonstrates that in this patient, a local production of IgM could be observed on day 2; on this day, "respiratory-membrane permeability" was low. On day 10 and 11, an increase of local IgM production was found. This was followed by an increase in "respiratory-membrane permeability" on day 16 and 17.

We conclude that the approach presented here opens up new possibilities with regard to the analysis of pathophysiological processes underlying asthma, chronic bronchitis and chronic obstructive airway disease.

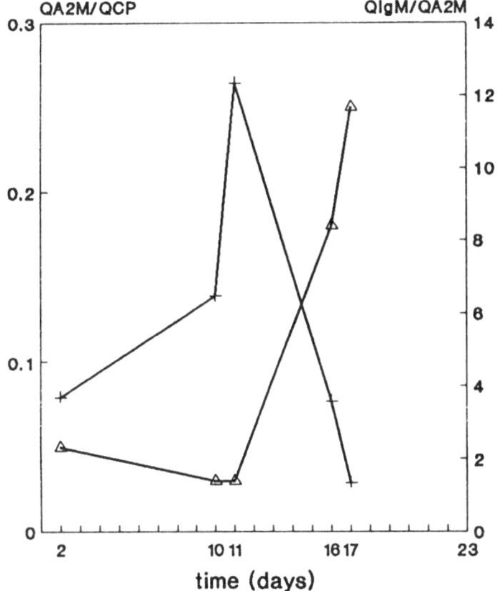

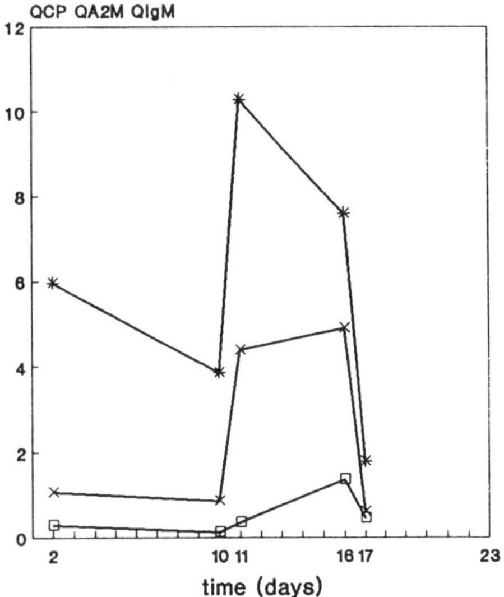

Figure 1. QCP,QA2M, QIgM, QA2M/QCP and QIgM/QA2M on different days after admission. During the period of sputum collection, the QA2M/QCP ratio remained stable on day 2, 10 and 11. On day 16 and 17 the QA2M/QCP ratio increased. The QIgM/QA2M had a value of 3.69 on day 2 and increased between day 2 and 10 and between day 10 and 11. On day 16 and 17, the QIgM/QA2M ratio had about the same value as on day 2. We conclude that local production of IgM occurred during day 2 and increased between day 2 and 10 and between day 10 and 11. The increase in the local production of IgM was followed by an increase in respiratory membrane permeability on day 16 and 17.
QCP, X-X; QA2M, - ; QIgM, *-*; QIgM/QA2M, +-+; QA2M/QCP,

ANTIBODIES IN SPUTUM

Antigens entering the body via the respiratory mucosal surface can stimulate secretory antibody formation in the local mucosal system. In many cases, the induction of IgA-antibodies in mucosal secretions is predominant and can occur when the serum antibody response is low. In allergic asthmatics, exposure to inhaled allergens results in a hyperergic state accompanied by the production of high amounts of local IgE antibodies. On the one hand, lack of tolerance to allergens entering the respiratory tract might - in the older chronic-asthmatic-bronchitis patient, too - be a factor, although allergic reactivity is diminished in these individuals as an age-related declining process. It may result in an upregulated local antibody response. On the other hand, as was mentioned above, the incidence of recurrent bacterial infections in the respiratory tract is markedly increased in chronic-asthmatic-bronchitis patients, suggesting a defect in the humoral defence mechanisms which may be due to a lack of local antibody formation or to an ineffectiveness on the part of the hyperergic humoral response.

Recently we demonstrated that infected COAD patients had significantly higher serum IgG and IgA antibody titres directed against well-defined immunocompetent outer-membrane proteins of Haemophilus influenzae (Groeneveld et al., 1990). The antibody titres in serum and SSF were determined by means of sensitive ELISA techniques. For each patient, the class-specific antibodies in serum had a specificity similar to the specificity of the antibodies in sputum. The specificity of IgA and IgG antibodies in sputum from infected and non-infected COAD patients was similar. Our results indicated that IgA antibodies were produced locally, in contrast to the IgG antibodies. The appearance or persistence of Haemophilus influenzae coincided with high levels of local antibody titres and specificity. From these studies, we concluded that COAD patients are infected with Haemophilus influenzae despite the presence of high local antibody concentrations directed against a variety of antigenic determinants of the infecting strain.

CONCLUSIONS: The findings reviewed in this paper support the hypothesis that local inflammation occurring in patients with chronic bronchitis and COAD causes a leakage of proteins from the blood into the respiratory lining fluid. Immunocompetent cells and secretory cells may be activated by this inflammatory process, and the products may even sustain the reaction.

Sequential studies, taking the inflammation-induced loss of size selectivity in the "respiratory membrane" into account, may afford insights into the extent of local inflammatory reactions in individual patients.

Acknowledgement: Ed A van de Graaf was supported by the Netherlands Asthma Foundation.

DISCUSSION

Persson.   I would like to suggest that the normal sieving function or size-selectivity of the epithelium to transudation of plasma proteins may be lost in patients where you have an ongoing inflammation in the airways.

Stockley.   I would like to comment on studies of α_2M and IgM. I think it is difficult to assess the effect of plasma leakage on these proteins since α_2M can be produced locally by macrophages and IgM is thought to be transported by a secretory component mediated transport across epithelial cells.

The evidence of local immunoglobulin memory relates to single exposure to viruses. In the patients you have studied the antigen is continually present and hence the local immunoglobulin response would persist. What is fascinating is why this response fails to remove the organisms.

Jansen. You are right about the production of α_2 macroglobulin by inflammatory cells, especially macrophages. However, this must be to a relatively low extent compared with what is coming from plasma. We have seen this in diseases like viral pneumonias where the leakage of α_2 macroglobulin is very much increased.

REFERENCES

Bell, D.Y., Haseman, J.A., Spock, A., McLennan, G., and Hook, G.E.R. (1981) Am. Rev. Respir. Dis. 124, 72-79.

Bowes, D., Clark, A.E., and Corrin, B. (1981) Thorax 36, 108-115.

Daniele, R.P., Altox, M.D., and Rowlands Jr, D.T. (1975) J. Clin. Invest. 56, 986-995.

Delacroix, D.L., Marchandise, F.X., Francis, C., and Sibille, Y. (1985) Am. Rev. Respir. Dis. 132, 829-835,

Gittlin, D., and Biassuci, A.. (1969) J. Clin. Invest. 48, 1433-1446.

Goodman, M.S., Link, D.W., Brown, W.R., and Nakane, P.K. (1981) Am. Rev. Respir. Dis. 123, 115-119.

Gorin, A.B., and Stewart, P.A., (1979) J. Appl. Physiol. 47, 1315-1324.

Groeneveld, K., Eijk P.P., Van Alphen L., Jansen H.M., and Zanen, H.C. (1990). Am. Rev. Respir. Dis. (in press).

Haimoto, H., Nagura, H., Imaizumi, M., Watanabe, K., and Iijima, S. (1984) Virchows Arch. 404, 369-380.

Hance, A.J., Saltini, C., and Crystal, R.C. (1988) Am. Rev. Resp. Dis. 137, 17-24.

Holter, J.F., Weiland, J.E., Pacht, E.R., Gadek, J.E., and Davis, W.B. (1986) J. Clin. Invest. 78, 1513-1522.

Laitinen L.A., Laitinen A., Widdicombe J. (1987) Am. Rev. Respir. Dis. 135, 67-70.

Lawrence, E.C., Blaese, R.M., Martin, R.R., and Stevens, P.M. (1978) J. Clin. Invest. 62, 832-835.

Masson, P.L., Heremans, J.F., Prignot, J.J., and Wauters, G. (1966) Thorax 21, 538-544.

Musher, D.M., Kubitschek, R.R., Crennan, J., and Baughm, R.E. (1983) Ann. Intern. Med. 99, 444-450.

Out T.A., Jansen H.M., Van Steenwijk R.P., De Nooijer M.J., Van de Graaf E.A., and Zuijderhoudt F.M.J. (1987) Clin. Chim. Acta. 165, 277-288.

Out, T.A., Van de Graaf, E.A., and Jansen, H.M. (1990) Eur. Resp. J., (in press).

Persson, G.G.A., and Erjefält, I. (1986) Acta Physiol. Scand. 126, 615-616.

Raphael, G.D., Jeney, E.V., Baraniuk, J.N., Kim, I., Meredith, S.D., and Kaliner, M.A. (1989) J. Clin. Invest. 84, 1528-1535.

Reichek, N., Lewin, E.B., Rhodem, D.L., Weaver, R.R., and
    Crutcher, J.C.(1970) Am. Rev. Resp. Dis. 101, 238-244.
Rossen, R.D., Morgan, C., Hsu, K.C., Butler, W.T., and Rose, H.M.
    (1968) J. Immunol. 100, 706-717.
Soutar, C.A. (1977) Thorax 32, 387-396.
Stockley, R.A., Mistry, M., Bradwell, A.R., and Burnett, D.
    (1979a) Thorax 34, 777-782.
Stockley, R.A., and Burnett, D. (1979b) Am. Rev. Respir. Dis
    111, 587-593.
Tourville, D.R., Adler, R.H., Bienenstock, J., and Tomasi, T.B.
    (1969) J. Exp. Med. 129, 411-429.
Van de Graaf, E.A., Kobesen, A., Out, T.A., Haaijman, J.J., and
    Jansen, H.M. (1988) Am. Rev. Respir. 137, A426.
Van de Graaf, E.A., Out, T.A., and Jansen, H.M. (1989) In:
    Glucocorticosteroids and Mechanisms of Asthma: Clinical and
    Experimental Aspects (F.E. Hargreave, J.C. Hogg, J.L. Malo,
    J.H. Toogood, Eds.), Excerpta Medica, Amsterdam, pp. 243-261.

21) A CRITICAL LOOK AT MUCUS MARKERS

J.G. Widdicombe

Department of Physiology, St George's Hospital Medical School,
Cranmer Terrace, London SW17 ORE, England

SUMMARY: Methods of collecting tracheobronchial secretions in
conditions such as chronic bronchitis are reviewed. The virtual
absence of such secretions in healthy lungs means that there is
no normal baseline for comparison. In addition, the inaccuracy
of most of the methods does not allow good quantitation of
secretory output. A large number of physical and chemical
analyses of secretions in many airways diseases does not point
to any variables which are specific for the diagnosis of chronic
bronchitis. This may be in part due to the contamination of
glandular secretion by epithelial secretion, transudation and
cellular debris. However, studies on mucus may be of value in
following the course of disease and its response in therapy.

INTRODUCTION

Chronic bronchitis is a disease characterized by an excessive
production of mucus and its expectoration. Indeed, the definition
of chronic bronchitis accepted by the Medical Research Council of
Great Britain (1965) is based almost entirely upon assessment of
increased expectoration. This definition was never satisfactory
for several reasons. There is no method of measuring with any
degree of accuracy the volume of submucosal gland secretion
produced in the lower respiratory tract in patients with chronic
bronchitis. Thus chronic bronchitis was defined as an increase in

a variable that cannot be accurately measured. Even if tracheo-bronchial secretion in disease could be quantitated, the resting secretion of mucus in healthy subjects is too small to be measured; estimates are of 50-150 ml per day, and even if these were accurate the volumes are too small to allow easy chemical or physical analysis in health (Richardson & Somerville, 1988). Thus there is no normal baseline on which to establish pathological increases in volume or changes in properties of secreted mucus.

Although pathological specimens from patients dying with chronic bronchitis show submucosal gland hypertrophy, this is of no value in premortem diagnosis. The Reid Index, the proportion of mucosa and submucosa occupied by submucosal glands in bronchial tissue (Lopez-Vidreiro & Reid, 1978) has in the past been used to assess chronic bronchitis in postmortem specimens. However, the Reid Index has no premortem value, and even post-mortem it is often difficult to distinguish between gland hyper-trophy and gland enlargement due to oedema.

Because of these difficulties in using mucus hypersecretion or gland hypertrophy for the diagnosis of chronic bronchitis, its recent definition by the American Thoracic Society (1987) omits any attempts to quantitate hypersecretion. In addition some patients with pathologically genuine chronic bronchitis may not have any detectable hypersecretion.

METHODS OF MUCUS COLLECTION

In spite of these reservations, it might be possible to collect lower airway mucus in patients with chronic bronchitis and to identify constituents or properties of value in diagnosis. The first problem is how to collect the mucus. Expectoration is the easiest method, and in the short term (possibly over minutes or less than an hour) a patient might be able to spit out all the mucus leaving the trachea (Bossi, 1988). However, in the longer term it is impossible to say how much mucus is swallowed, so quantitation is not accurate. In addition, expectoration is contaminated to an unknown amount by sputum, which will change its chemical and physical properties. To some extent the problem of contamination with saliva can be met by "protective expectoration" in which saliva is prevented from reaching the expectorate (Puchelle et al., 1984). This method may be valuable for short-term collection of mucus.

The most direct method for collecting tracheobronchial mucus is by aspiration either through a bronchoscope or via the transtracheal route (Bossi, 1988). The latter may be inappropriate for routine use. As explained above, if you can aspirate mucus then its production is probably "pathological", since virtually none is produced in health. Aspiration of mucus may be valuable if a bronchoscope has to be passed for other reasons, but otherwise it probably has few advantages over collection of sputum. In addition, the procedures leading up to aspiration, including the use of sedatives, and possible atropinic drugs and local anaesthesia, may change the nature of the aspirate in unidentifiable ways.

If there is not enough mucus to be aspirated, bronchial washings may provide a source of secretions. The extent to which the washing medium itself changes the nature of the secretions is not clear, and will be discussed later.

A final consideration is that, if one is to search for chemical markers for chronic bronchitis in airway secretions, the use of tissue explants or cell cultures may be a valuable research tool (van Scott et al., 1986). Bronchial explants and cell cultures from patients with chronic bronchitis are easy to obtain, since they frequently have lung resection for carcinoma. Comparison can be made between the secretions from these explants and cells with those from more healthy resected lung.

SOURCES OF MUCUS SECRETIONS

However collected, the secretions probably are derived from two sources: the periciliary fluid and submucosal gland secretions. There have been extensive studies on the control of output and chemistry of both types of secretion (Marin, 1986; Richardson & Somerville, 1988; Widdicombe, 1989). It is usually assumed that the periciliary fluid is a liquid of low viscosity and probably low in glycoprotein content, whereas the gland secretion lying on the tips of the cilia is highly viscous and rich in glycoprotein. Although the macromolecular distinction between the two liquids may be valid, it is not clear to what extent small solutes can diffuse in and out of the two layers. In particular, the control of periciliary fluid is thought to be mainly a function of epithelial ciliated cells, and if this secretion is changed it may interact with the secretions from submucosal glands. Collected sputum is frequently centrifuged do divide it into sol and gel layers, and it is often assumed that these correspond to periciliary and glandular secretory liquids. This assumption has never been justified.

PHYSICAL ANALYSIS OF SECRETIONS

There have been many studies of the rheology of lower airway secretions, often measuring separately the viscosity and elasticity of the liquids (Davis, 1988). It is probably true to say that such physical analyses have never shown a clear distinction between the secretions in chronic bronchitis and those in other lung diseases. As explained already, there is no way in which pathological secretions can be compared with healthy ones, since the latter are too scanty for analysis. At a diagnostic tool, mucus rheology largely fails because the major factor affecting rheology is the contamination of the mucus by substances from other sources (Boat & Matthews, 1973). Its visco-elasticity is profoundly influenced, for example, by DNA, which is present whenever infection and cell destruction take place. Other factors that change rheology are the amount of albumin present, which is increased by epithelial transudation, and the amount and types of phospholipids (Widdicombe, 1987). The last are derived both from alveolar surfactant and from cell damage in the airways. Infection and cell damage are so common in the vast majority of chronic airway diseases as to invalidate rheology as a diagnostic tool in the absence of these complications.

A more instructive physical variable to measure might be the adhesiveness of mucus, and in-vitro methods have been developed to study this (Puchelle & Zahm, 1988). However, the in-vitro adhesivity or "tackiness" of mucus is probably only of indirect significance (Lopez-Vidreiro, 1988). What is more important is the in-situ adhesiveness of the mucus to airway epithelium, especially when the latter has been damaged by disease or when there is transudation of serum proteins that change the adhesiveness of the mucus to tissue. The question of mucus adhesiveness in vivo is an important one which has received insufficient study.

CHEMICAL ANALYSES OF SECRETION

Tracheobronchial secretions contain a large number of components (Boat & Cheng, 1980; Moretti, 1988; Richardson & Somerville, 1988). Some of these are indicators of cell destruction, such as DNA and neutral lipids including cholesterol. Others, such as mucoglycoproteins, might be more specific for gland secretions and, if their chemical constitution could be shown to be abnormal in chronic bronchitis compared with other diseases, might have diagnostic value. In practice, however, such chemical analysis has little diagnostic value (Lopez-Vidreiro & Reid, 1978; Boat & Cheng, 1980.

Total macromolecules: One of the simplest tests for total macro-molecules in secretions is to measure their dry weight. One per cent of body fluids consist of electrolytes and small solutes, and any excess over one per cent approximately represents macro-molecules (Lusuardi & Donner, 1988). It would include all the macromolecules mentioned below. This measure would be complicated by any evaporation from the secretions, by contamination with cell debris, and in any event has not been correlated with particular lung diseases.

Mucoglycoproteins: Full mucoglycoprotein analysis is highly complex, and more appropriate as a research tool than in clinical diagnosis. The mucoglycoproteins have molecular weights up to 15 x 10^6 Da, and their analysis is formidable (Kaliner et al., 1986; Creeth, 1987). Even the measurement to the total amount of mucoglycoprotein in secretions is difficult. Many methods will confuse them with proteoglycans (see below).

Measurement of total hexoses in secretions is simple, and since mucoglycoproteins have a higher hexose content than other glycosylated proteins, this may give an indication of their content. However, it is more informative to measure specific hexoses that label mucoglycoproteins, in particular fucose. Much experimental work has shown that this is a good index of glandular mucoglycoprotein secretion, although it may not have diagnostic value in airways diseases. Similarly, the ratio of acid to neutral mucoglycoproteins increases in experimental chronic bronchitis in animals, and there is some indication that it may be high in human chronic bronchitis (Lopez-Vidreiro & Reid, 1978). There are relatively easy ways of determining this ratio, such as the use of acid and neutral dyes with colorimetric analysis. However, once again such methods seem to lack diagnostic value in human disease. Measurement of sulphate or sialic acid content also indicates the amount of acid mucoglycoprotein (Lusuardi & Donner, 1988), but the ratio of the latter to the neutral macromolecules does not seem to give specific information about chronic bronchitis.

Use of monoclonal antibodies: A potentially more valuable method is to analyze amounts of mucus glycoprotein using monoclonal antibodies. Much research on this aspect is currently being performed, and the availability of appropriate monoclonal antibodies may provide a useful tool for measuring the amount of secretory mucoglycoprotein in the airways (Basbaum et al., 1986).

Whether this method will also have diagnostic value remains to be determined.

Other glycosylated proteins: The airway epithelium, probably the ciliated cells, can secrete proteoglycans in response to irritation, damage and possibly inflammatory mediators (Richardson & Somerville, 1988). Methods which assess total glycosylated proteins, or total sugar content, will not distinguish between proteoglycans and mucoglycoproteins. Immunoglobulins are also hexose-rich and their presence could cause confusion.

Specific markers: Specific markers for submucosal gland secretion include compounds such as lysozyme, lactoferrin and some immunoglobulins, all of which are produced by cells in serous acini (Boat & Cheng, 1980; Olivieri & Mori, 1988). The ratio of these specific markers to total mucoglycoprotein might indicate whether or not the main secretion is from serous or mucous acini.

Lipids: Some of the most careful chemical analyses of tracheobronchial secretions have been on the lipid contents, in the hope that this method would provide specific markers for lung diseases (Widdicombe, 1987). However, the balance of lipid contents (including neutral lipids, free fatty acids, phospholipids from alveoli and airways, and triglycerides) has given values of such enormous diversity with various conditions of collection and in various lung diseases, that their analysis has no diagnostic value. It is mentioned to give an example of the great variability of secretory chemistry found with different methods and in different diseases.

Electrolytes: It is sometimes assumed that the electrolyte composition of airway surface liquid is close to that of interstitial fluid. Recent studies show that this is not correct and that, at least in ferrets and probably dogs, tracheobronchial airway surface liquid is hypertonic, due to a high content of sodium and chloride, and in addition has high concentrations of potassium and calcium (Boucher et al., 1981; Robinson et al., 1989,; Widdicombe, 1989). It has a relatively low pH (under 7.0) which seems to be autoregulated in the presence of external changes in pH. The cause of these unusual ionic compositions presumably resides in the secretory mechanisms of the epithelium. The same epithelium can actively transport albumin from interstitium into lumen.

These results are significant for several reasons. They indicate that the use of "physiological saline" for lavage may be physiologically undesirable, in that it introduces an unusual medium. In terms of airways diseases, corresponding values for electrolytes in airway surface liquid have not been reported. However, one might expect them to change in conditions where airway epithelium is damaged or destroyed. Whether or not such changes would be sufficiently large to have diagnostic value cannot be said at present, and in any event as indicated earlier there are no convenient non-invasive ways to collect airway surface liquid.

CONCLUSION: In spite of extensive research on the physical and chemical properties of tracheobronchial secretions, these properties have not been defined in ways that have clear diagnostic value for lung diseases such as chronic bronchitis. This is partly because a major factor determining the physics and chemistry of airway secretions is the presence of infection and tissue damage, which will be common to most chronic lung diseases and also highly variable between them. In addition, the paucity of secretions in healthy airways does not provide an adequate normal baseline. However, even if studies on the properties of mucus have little diagnostic value in chronic bronchitis, they may be informative in identifying the development of the disease and the patient's response to therapy.

DISCUSSION

Brattsand. How rapid may the secretion of albumin into the airway lumen be? Does it originate from the submucosal plexus or from the glands?

Widdicombe. We have measured secretion of albumin over periods of 15 min or longer, so we don't know the minimum time. Since we can observe secretion into lumen of the rabbit trachea, a species that lacks submucosal glands, we believe that the transport is not glandular but is across the epithelium.

Brattsand. Do you have evidences for active secretion of also other macromolecules?

Widdicombe. We have only looked at dextrans (70000 and 9000 kDa) which are transported far more slowly than is albumin, and we are sure that they are transported passively.

Arborelius. There are some reports from the sixties, that serum albumin introduced into the lungs of dogs passes to the blood with a half-time of about 30 minutes. The process must be active as it occurs also against concentrations.

Widdicombe. In our model, albumin was transported several times faster from interstitium to lumen than either of the dextrans, suggesting that it is being transported actively. There are publications showing that albumin can be actively transported from lumen to interstitium in the bullfrog alveolar wass and the dog bronchial lumen. Therefore, it is possible that the transport can be bidirectional, the effective direction depending on the site and the experimental conditions.

Pride. Presumably samples of the airway surface liquid are from large airways. Are there any indications this varies in different sized airways?

Widdicombe. We have only looked at the ferret trachea. Different size airways have different ion-pumping systems and transepithelial potential differences, so the composition of airway surface liquid may also be different.

REFERENCES

American Thoracic Society. (1987) Am. Rev. Respir. Dis. 136, 225-244.

Basbaum, C.B., Chow, A., Macher, B.A., Finkbeiner, W.E., Vessiere, D., and Forsberg, L.S. (1986) Arch. Biochem. Biophys. 249, 363-373.

Boat, T.F., and Cheng, P.W. (1980) Fec. Proc. 39, 3067-3074.

Boat, T.F., and Matthews, L.V. (1973) In: Sputum, Fundamentals and Clinical Pathology (M.J. Dulfano, Ed), Charles C. Thomas, Springfield, IL, pp. 243-273.

Bossi, R. (1988) In: Methods in Bronchial Mucology (P.C. Braga and L. Allegra, Eds), Raven Press, New York, pp. 13-20.

Boucher, R.C., Stutts, M.J., Bromberg, P.A., and Gatzy, J.T. (1981) J.Appl. Physiol. 50, 613-620.

Creeth, J.M. (1978) Br. Med. Bull. 34, 17-24.

Davis, S.S. (1988) In: Methods in Bronchial Mucology (P.C. Braga and L. Allegra, Eds), Raven Press, New York, pp. 33-49.

Kaliner, M., Shelhamer, J.H., Borson, B., Nadel, J., Patow, C., and Marom, Z. (1986) Am. Rev. Respir. Dis. 134, 612-621.

Lopez-Vidreiro, M.T. (1988) In: Methods in Bronchial Mucology (P.C. Braga and L. Allegra, Eds), Raven Press, New York, pp. 141-152.

Lopez-Vidreiro, M.T., and Reid, L. (1978) Br. Med. Bull. 34, 63-74.

Lusuardi, M., and Donner, C.F. (1988) In: Methods in Bronchial Mucology (P.C. Braga and L. Allegra, Eds), Raven press, New York, pp. 155-169).

Marin, M.G. (1986) Pharmacol. Rev. 38, 273-289.

Medical Research Council. (1965) Lancet ii, 775-779.

Moretti, M. (1988) In: Methods in Bronchial Mucology (P.C. Braga and L. Allegra, Eds), Raven Press, New York, pp. 171-188.

Olivieri, D., and Mori, P.A. (1988) Ibid, pp. 201-208.

Puchelle, E., Tournier, J.M., Zahm, J.M., and Sadoul, P. (1984) J. Lab. Clin. Med 103, 347-353.

Puchelle, E., and Zahm, J.M. (1988) In: Methods in Bronchial Mucology (P.C. Braga and L. Allegra, Eds), Raven Press, New York, pp. 135-139.

Richardson, P.S., and Somerville, M. (1988) In: Asthma: Basic Mechanisms and Clinical Management (P.J. Barnes, I.W. Rodger and N.C. Thomson, Eds), Acadmic Press, London, pp. 163-186.

Robinson, N.P., Kyle, H., Webber, S.E., and Widdicombe, J.G. (1989) J. Appl. Physiol. 66, 2129-2135.

Van Scott, M.R., Yankaskas, J.R., and Boucher, R.C. (1986) Exp. Lung Res. 11, 75-94.

Widdicombe, J.G. (1987) Eur. J. Respir. Dis. 71 (suppl 153), 197-204.

Widdicombe, J.G. (1989) Eur. Respir. J. 2, 107-115.

Widdicombe, J.H. (1988) In: Methods in Bronchial Mucology (P.C. Braga and L. Allegra, Eds), Raven Press, New York, pp. 291-302.

22) POINTS OF IMPORTANCE IN LONG TERM INTERVENTION STUDIES IN CB/COAD

C.G Löfdahl, S. Larsson, and B.E. Skoogh

Department of Pulmonary Medicine, Renströmska Hospital, Gothenburg University, Gothenburg, Sweden.

Chronic obstructive airways disease (COAD) has a high prevalence in all westernized countries, often with rates up to 10 % of the population in people over 50 years of age (Fletcher, 1976; Feinleib, 1989; Manfreda, 1989). The disease also has a severe prognosis, more severe than asthma (Burrows, 1969; 1987; 1989; Anthonisen, 1986; 1989).

Smoking cessation has earlier been shown to improve prognosis. Some studies have also shown that oxygen therapy improves the prognosis in severe cases of COAD (Nocturnal Oxygen Therapy Trial group, 1980; Medical Research council working party, 1981). More recently retrospective studies have indicated that glucocorticoids might improve the outcome in patients with COAD (Postma, 1985; 1988). These observations have initiated a further interest in intervention studies in chronic obstructive airways disease, and a special interest has been focused to the question whether pharmacological treatment might improve the prognosis of the disease. This chapter summaries part of the current discussion and describes some points considered relevant in planning an intervention study in COAD.

Such a study will most likely need many patients, and,

therefore, a multicenter trial will be necessary. The further discussion will deal with the choice of effect parameters, selection of patients, duration of study and number of patients needed, including an evaluation of statistical power of such a study. Furthermore, this chapter will deal with some practical aspects and ethical considerations for a long term intervention study in COAD.

EFFECT PARAMETERS

Mortality, the ultimate parameter, is increased in COAD. In studies of long-term oxygen treatment in COAD the mortality rate has been a discriminative effect parameter (Nocturnal Oxygen Therapy Trial group, 1980; Medical Research council working party, 1981). The patients in need of oxygen are, however, in a late phase of their disease associated with a high mortality rate. Mortality figures can only be expected to be discriminative in intervention studies on patients with very severe chronic airflow limitation, for instance FEV_1 less than 30 % predicted (Anthonisen, 1989). This implies that mortality figures will have a low discriminative value for intervention studies in earlier phases of COAD. As airways obstruction in COAD is to a large extent irreversible, the expected long-term effect of a beneficial pharmacologic intervention will be prevention of further deterioration of airways obstruction, rather than an actual improvement. Consequently, an intervention ought to be done in an early phase of the disease. This consideration invalidates mortality as an effect parameter and calls for measures of airway patency like FEV_1. Moreover, the initial value of FEV_1 correlates well with later mortality and is therefore a good indicator of the future prognosis of the disease (Anthonisen, 1989).

The annual decline of FEV_1 is increased in COAD, and patients with the most severe prognosis have the most rapid decline of FEV_1 (Fletcher, 1976; Anthonisen, 1989; Burrows, 1989). Smoking cessation has been proved to decrease the decline per year

(Fletcher, 1976), and thereby improve the prognosis. Thus, this measure has been shown to have a discriminative power in long-term studies of COAD.

To plan long-term studies of COAD it is important to know the variation of the decline in various studies. Several studies have evaluated the annual decline of FEV_1 in populations with different types of obstructive airways disease. In Fletcher's study in patients with COAD, the mean annual decline in moderate smokers (less than 15 cig./day) was 63 ml/year, whereas heavy smokers (more than 15 cig./day) showed a decrease of 78 ml/year (Fletcher, 1976). After smoking cessation, the decline was the same as in healthy smokers (36 ml/year). Burrows has in several studies from Arizona and Chicago shown that the mean annual decline of FEV_1 in COAD was 70 ml/year, whereas patients with asthmatic bronchitis only had a mean annual decline of 5 ml/year (Burrows, 1969; 1989; Burrows et al., 1987). In Anthonisen's material of COAD patients from Canada, the mean decline/year was 48 ml. The most pronounced decline was in patients with baseline FEV_1 40-49 % predicted, whereas only about 35 ml/year was lost if baseline FEV1 ≥50 % predicted.

With these figures as a background we have in the further discussion stated that a clinically significant reduction due to a pharmacologic intervention is a decreased decline of 20 ml/year as measured by FEV_1.

EXACERBATIONS OF CHRONIC BRONCHITIS

Patients with COAD also frequently suffer from chronic bronchitis. In patients with chronic bronchitis, exacerbations is a factor of importance for quality of life and working capacity (Boman et al., 1983). It has been shown that the number of exacerbations can be reduced by pharmacological intervention in chronic bronchitis. N-acetylcystein significantly reduced the number of exacerbations in patients with chronic bronchitis and mild to moderate airways obstruction (Boman et al., 1983). To evaluate exacerbations questionnaires including questions concerning sputum quality and other respiratory symptoms are used. As exacerbations occur rather infrequently, long follow up periods and rather big numbers of patients are needed.

In long-term trials of obstructive airways disease other parameters than exacerbation frequency could be used, such as specific symptom scores. However, to our knowledge, no good evaluation of symptom scores have been done in long-term trials, with the exception of the questionnaires evaluating infectious exacerbations. General quality of life-questionnaires have to some extent been used in the evaluation of COAD. The SIP-instrument (Sickness Impact Profile) was tried in the NOTT-study of oxygen therapy in COAD (Nocturnal Oxygen Therapy Trial group, 1980). It was, however, not possible to show any effect of oxygen treatment on this quality of life measurement. Others have started to use the instrument in less severely ill patients, but at this stage it is difficult to recommend it for general use. Furthermore, these questionnaires are very laborious, why it is difficult to use them in a large multicenter trial.

Other parameters, such as measurement of mucociliary clearance, studies of cellular markers of inflammation achieved from broncho-alveolar lavage, measurement of bronchial hyper-responsiveness could possibly give valuable information in a study of long term intervention in COAD. However, they are rather laborious methods, and difficult to standardize for use in a multicenter study.

Summarizing, the primary effect parameter to be used in long term intervention studies in COAD seems to be the annual decline of FEV_1, and a possible secondary parameter could be the exacerbation rate of infections.

PATIENT SELECTION

The diagnosis of COAD should be established in current or possibly former smokers with airway obstruction. Bronchial asthma should be excluded with a high probability. The smoking history should be regular smoking for at least 10 years. As the most important effect parameter is the decline in FEV_1, only patients with an increased decline rate are of interest. The ideal situation would be to select patients who have shown a substantial annual decline of FEV_1 during a prolonged time period. However, then a large population need to be screened during a long time. An alternative method could be to choose patients of relatively young age with already a clearly decreased FEV_1. A suggestion would be patients between 30 and 60 years of age with a post bronchodilator FEV_1 between e.g. 45 and 75 % of predicted normal value. Lower values might indicate a risk of developing respiratory insufficiency during the trial period.

To exclude bronchial asthma patients with a history of asthma, a reversibility above 20 % or with signs of atopy should be excluded. If the number of exacerbations of infections is used as an effect parameter, patients with sputum problems who are known to have a certain number of infectious exacerbations per year should be included.

NUMBER OF PATIENTS

To study the annual decline of FEV_1 in a double blind placebo controlled study estimations of the variance within and between patients must be done. The within patient variation is dependent on the number of measurements per year and also the duration of the study. From a long term study in industrial workers (Berry, 1974) the within patient variation was 120 ml/year and the between patient variation 40 ml/year. In another material (Bates, 1989) the within patient variation was 190 ml/year and the between patient variation the same as in previous material. On a basis of four measurements per year during 3 years, the estimation of the total standard deviation is less than 70 ml/year.

If the clinically significant effect is a reduction by 20 ml/year of the annual decline of FEV_1, that comprises 29 % of the standard deviation. To achieve a power of 80 % in a three year study, a total number of 350 patients divided into two groups is needed. If instead the duration of the study is two years, still with four measurements per year, the number of patients has to be 460 to achieve 80 % power in the trial.

A recommendation, therefore, could be to follow 350 patients during 3 years with 4 FEV_1 measurements per year. With that choice of trial size it can be calculated that if the placebo-treated group has 25 % higher frequency of exacerbations a mean of about 2 exacerbations per year and patient is needed in the placebo treated group. If the frequency is 50 % higher in the placebo treated group, a mean of 0.7 exacerbations per patient and year is needed.

As patients with COAD not always show both a decrease of FEV_1 and a high exacerbation rate it will be difficult to select patients with a low FEV_1 and concomitantly such a high frequency of exacerbations. Therefore, we believe it will not be possible to include exacerbation rate as a parameter in a trial of this kind. To evaluate the question of exacerbations a separate study has to be done with a different patient selection.

SMOKING HABITS

As COAD is a disease that is mainly dependent on smoking habits, and as the annual decline of FEV_1 is correlated to the number of cigarettes smoked, it is important how smoking is handled during a trial of this disease (Fletcher, 1976). We think it would be unethical to study these patients without giving them explicit advice and help to quit smoking. It could also blur the result if a great number of the patients change their smoking habits during the trial. Therefore, we think it is important to have a run-in period, where patients have taken part in a smoking cessation program. Only patients who are not able to quit smoking are then included in the trial.

REFERENCES

Anthonisen, N.R. (1989) Am. Rev. Respir. Dis. <u>140</u> (3:2), 95-99.

Anthonisen, N.R., and Hodgkin, J.E. Am. Rev. Respir. Dis. (1986) <u>133</u>, 14-20.

Bates, D. (1989) Ed. Respiratory Function in Disease, 3rd Ed., WB Saunders Co., Philadelphia.

Berry, G. (1974) Bull. Physio-path. Resp. <u>10</u>, 643-655.

Boman, G., Backer, U., Larsson, S., Melander, B., and Wahlander, L. (1983) Eur. Respir. Dis. <u>64</u>, 405-412.

Burrows, B. (1989) Am. Rev. Respir. Dis. <u>140</u> (3:2), 92-94.

Burrows, B., Traver, G.A., and Cline, M.G. (1987) N. Engl. J. Med. <u>317</u>, 1309-1314.

Burrows, B.E.R. (1969) N. Engl. J. Med. <u>280</u>, 397-404.

Feinleib, M., Collins, J.G., Delozier, J.E., Pokras, R., and Chevarley, F.M. (1989) Am. Rev. Respir. Dis. <u>140</u> (3:2), 9-18.

Fletcher, C., Tinker, C., and Speizer, F.E. (1976) London: Oxford University Press,

Manfreda, J., and Litven, W. (1989) Am. Rev. Respir. Dis. <u>140</u> (3:2), 19-26.

Medical Research Council Working Party. (1981) Lancet <u>1</u>, 681-686.

Nocturnal Oxygen Therapy Trial Group. (1980) Ann. Intern. Med. <u>93</u>, 391-398.

Postma, D.S., Steenhuis, E.J., and Sluiter, H.J. (1988) Eur. Respir. J. <u>1</u>, 22-26.

Postma, D.S., van der Weele, L.T., and Sluiter H.J. (1985) Eur. J. Respir. Dis. <u>67</u>, 56-64.

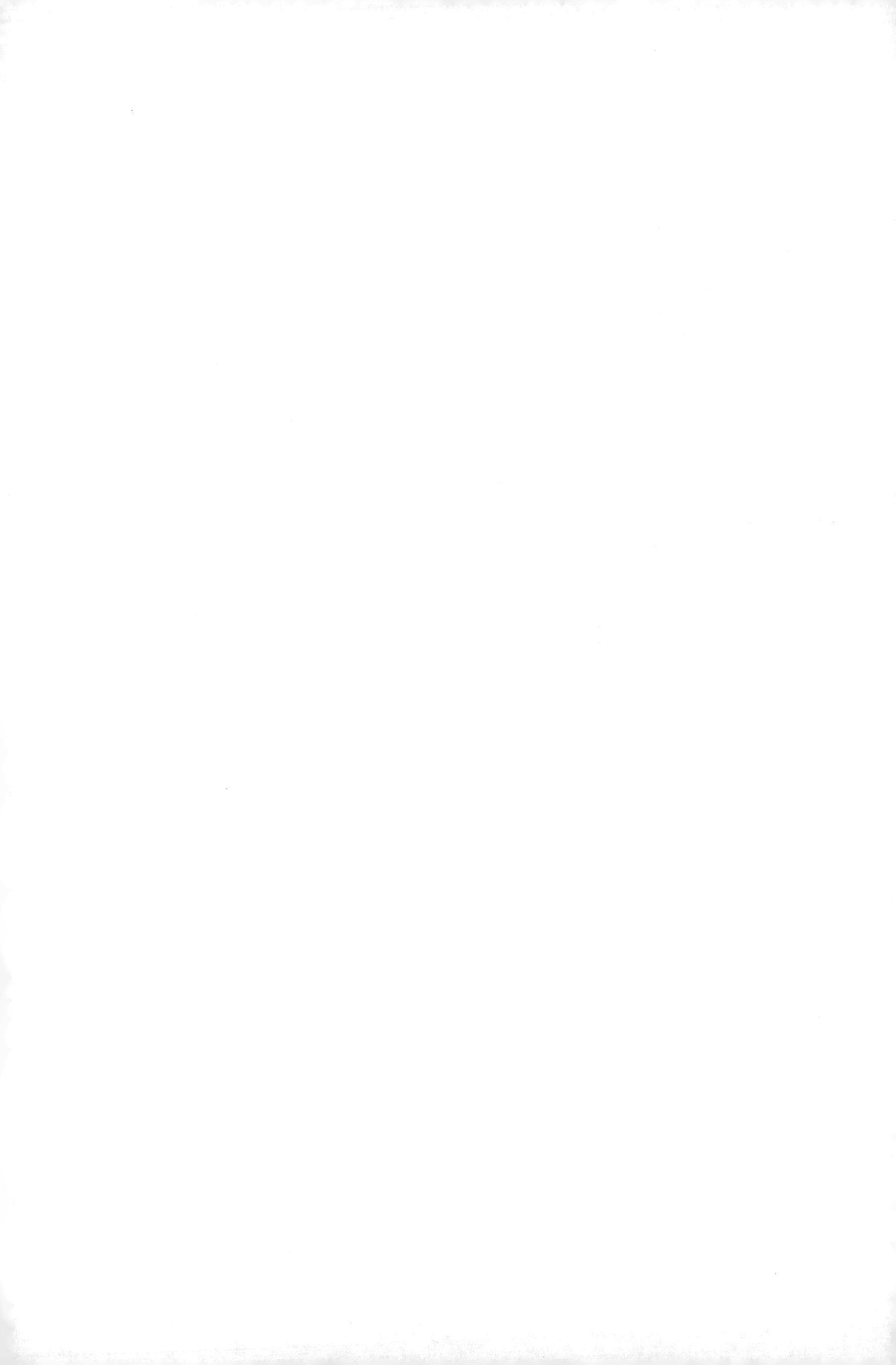

23) WHICH MARKERS OF INFLAMMATION SHOULD BE USED IN THERAPEUTIC INTERVENTION STUDIES OF CB/COAD?

P. Venge[1], R.Brattsand[2], L.A. Laitinen[3], and C.G.A. Persson[4]

[1]Laboratory for Inflammation Research, Department of Clinical Chemistry, University Hospital, S-751 85 Uppsala, Sweden, [2]Laboratory of Pharmacology, AB Draco, Lund, Sweden, [3]Department of Explorative Clinical Research, AB Draco, Lund, Sweden, [4]Department of Clinical Pharmacology, University of Lund, Lund, Sweden.

SAMPLES

Before discussing the particular indices, it is important to consider the possibilities of getting proper samples of tracheo-bronchial surface liquids and tissue. Sputum, bronchial lavage liquids, and biopsies are important samples and provide complementary information (see Table I). It was agreed that bronchial lavage and, particularly, bronchial biopsy studies can only be performed in a few, highly specialized centers.

Table I. Some characteristics of sputa, bronchial lavage liquids and biopsies in studies of bronchial diseases.

Sputum

+ Non-invasive

+ Airway specific, but saliva contaminates

contd/

+ Can be obtained frequently in select patients

+ Actual mucosal surface concentrations of solutes may approximately be determined

- Cannot be obtained in healthy subjects or in many patients because of poor and variable production

- Yield cannot readily be increased: secretagogues need validation

- Its cell content needs validation

- Baseline variations because the time period for production is unknown

- The producing airway is not identified

- Indices in sol- and gel-phases, respectively, need validation

Bronchial lavage

+ Harvests cells for cell counts and select functional studies

+ Can be carried out in both healthy subjects and patients (also those without any sputum production)

+ Defined time point sampling is obtained

- The sampled material has accumulated on the mucosa for an unknown period of time

- Alveolar lining material may contaminate the sampled bronchial material or may dominate the sample if large volume lavages are used.

- Invasive; requires systemic and topical medication; may induce a degree of trauma in the airways

- Cannot be performed frequently

- Solute indices of the airways are diluted to an unknown extent; data preferably presented in the raw form as well as corrected for denominators of dilution

- The importance of specific examination of mucus lumps in the lavage liquid needs validation

Bronchial biopsy

+ Represents material from actual localization of disease, although from a small area

contd/

+ May be processed for several different methods (light microscopy, transmission electron microscopy, scanning electron microscopy, immunohistochemistry, biochemistry, tissue cultures etc.)

+ Provides quantitative information on tissue pathology at cellular and subgross histology levels

- Presently, little reference material is available both from normal subjects and disease groups

- Specimens are relatively small and need validation in correlation to the airways as a whole

- Invasive; requires systemic and topical medication; induces a degree of trauma in the airways

- Cannot be performed frequently; difficult to perform in normal subjects

- Special skill required to properly master the technique

INDICES

During the meeting an abundance of indices of inflammation in CB and COAD was presented (Table II). By monitoring some of these markers it might be possible to elucidate whether or not an intervention alters the disease activity in a desired direction. The seasonal variation in some functions of inflammatory cells may necessitate parallel groups design in such studies. For practical reasons, only a selection of these indices may be monitored in therapeutic intervention studies of CB and COAD. The purpose of this discussion was, therefore, to identify the most relevant and manageable indices.

The number of blood cells should be counted in all patients. Sputum cells may well be counted, but it was pointed out that the technique of counting cells in sputum is not widely established. The reproducibility in the sputum cell counting needs validation. Subtyping of cells, based on identification of specific membrane molecules, was discussed but not recommended.

Analysis of albumin (and fibrinogen) as indicators of plasma exudation/transudation were recommended, whereas other plasma proteins such as protease inhibitors and immunoglobulins could be determined in a select subgroup of patients.

Table II. Potentially important inflammatory indices in blood, sputum, bronchial lavage liquids and biopsies obtained from patients with CB and COAD.

1.   Cell numbers and subpopulations.

2.   Markers of the activity of specific cells such as:

    - ECP for eosinophils
    - MPO for neutrophils
    - Lysozyme for macrophages
    - Tryptase for mast cells
    - Hyaluronic acid for fibroblasts
    - TNF, interleukins for macrophages, T-lymphocytes and other cells
    - Lactoferrin for submucosal glands

3.   Plasma tracers: albumin, fibrinogen, immunoglobulins etc

4.   Plasma-derived active factors: proteases, bradykinins

5.   Mucus markers: secretory IgA etc

6.   Functional activities of:

    - monocytes/macrophages
    - neutrophils

7.   Chemotactic activities

8.   Others

Specific extracellular markers of inflammatory cell activity are also suited for determination in all available material: ECP (eosinophil cationic protein) as a marker of eosinophil involvement and myeloperoxidase (MPO) as a marker of the neutrophils. In blood, but not in sputum or lung lavage fluids, lysozyme is a good indicator of macrophage involvement. In sputum, after ultracentrifugation or sonication, ECP and possibly MPO may be used to estimate the number of eosinophils and neutrophils more accurately than the counting of these cells. The measurement of other cell markers such as tryptase from mast cells, hyaluronic acid from fibroblasts, TNF and various interleukins from monocytes/macrophages, T-lymphocytes and other cells was not recommended. More data are required to prove that these markers are meaningful. Similarly, markers of glandular activity, such as lactoferrin, were not thought to be important. It is likely that the exacerbations in CB are associated with the accumulation of inflammatory cells in the lung. Hence, it might be of interest to measure the local generation of chemotactic signals. Indeed, this was recommended to be performed routinely in sputum and also in lung lavage fluids when available.

Monitoring of neutrophil and monocyte functions in blood should be included but has to be restricted to a small subgroup of patients since it requires close access to a highly specialized laboratory. From available data it seems that the oxidative metabolism, the phagocytosing and secretory capacity of these two cell types are the most relevant function to assess. In addition, the chemotactic responsiveness of the neutrophils is of importance. In the centers where it is feasible, the phagocytosis, the secretory functions and the oxidative metabolism of alveolar macrophages should be examined.

Table III summarizes our attempts at consensus. Basically, it involves the measurements in sputum and blood of cells and of components which could be stored in a freezer for later analyses. BAL and BL and the functional testing of cellular activities in BAL and BL material can be carried out only in highly specialized centers.

Table III. Consensus on routine (1-4) and specialized center (5-7) work.

1. Cell numbers in blood and sputum.

2. Plasma proteins such as albumin and fibrinogen in blood and sputum.

3. Cell markers ECP, Lysozyme and MPO in serum/plasma.

4. Chemotactic activity, ECP and MPO in sputum, the latter two as markers of eosinophils and neutrophil numbers.

5. As above (1-4) but also in BAL- and BL-liquids.

contd/

6. Measuring monocyte/macrophage activity of cells obtained from blood and BAL.

7. Neutrophil activity measurements with cells from blood.

DRUGS

With the exception of thiols and antibiotics, the major drugs now used for the treatment of CB/COAD are those primarily developed for combatting asthma. The drugs range from bronchodilators represented by antimuscarinics, over β_2-agonists and xanthines, which have both bronchodilating and other airway protective effects, to the anti-inflammatory glucocorticoids. Inhalant glucocorticoids such as beclomethasone dipropionate and, more recently, budesonide, with a high degree of airway specificity are available. There have also been significant developments in multidose inhaler devices. The pure glucocorticoid drug powder can now be conveniently delivered to the bronchi without irritating freons or carrier substances. Hence, the possibilities for topical inhibition of airway inflammation have improved markedly.

The glucocorticoid drugs may affect many of the inflammatory indices discussed above, but critical examination of these actions in airway disease remains to be carried out. Furthermore, it is not known to what extent anti-inflammatory actions of inhaled glucocorticoids may affect the long term progress of CB/COAD.